SURGERY – PROCEDURES, COMPLICATIONS, AND RESULTS

HANDBOOK OF SURGICAL PROCEDURES

SURGERY – PROCEDURES, COMPLICATIONS, AND RESULTS

Additional books and e-books in this series can be found on Nova's website under the Series tab.

SURGERY – PROCEDURES, COMPLICATIONS, AND RESULTS

HANDBOOK OF SURGICAL PROCEDURES

HEATHER GILBERT
EDITOR

nova
Medicine & Health
New York

Additional color graphics may be available in the e-book version of this book.

Library of Congress Cataloging-in-Publication Data

ISBN: 978-1-53614-580-9
Library of Congress Control Number: 2018960106

Published by Nova Science Publishers, Inc. † New York

CONTENTS

PREFACE

In this compilation, the authors begin with a focus on the indications for surgery in hepatocarcinoma and how to perform a liver resection. Long-term outcomes and different theories on the causes of recurrence after resection are also discussed.

Most patients with hepatocarcinoma have underlying chronic liver disease and are thus at high risk for development of postoperative complications, which can sometimes be fatal. The authors propose that we may be able to prolong the overall survival of patients by using laparoscopic liver resection as a powerful local therapy, which can be applied repeatedly with minimal deterioration of liver function.

Bronchoscopy has become an important procedure for diagnostic and therapeutic purposes, particularly in the context of lung cancer. As such, the medical and surgical advances in bronchoscopy are described herein.

Post-operative pancreatic fistula is one of the most dreaded complications in any pancreatic operation given its associated morbidity and mortality. This collection examines how the amylase-rich fluid can cause inflammation, become infected, or cause serious bleeding from neighboring vasculature.

The authors go on to discuss cystic fibrosis, the most common life-threatening autosomal recessive disorder affecting Caucasians. The indications of endoscopic sinus surgery in cystic fibrosis patients are discussed, drawing from personal experience in the diagnosis and treatment of cystic fibrosis-related sinus disorders.

Following this, the origins of functional sinus surgery as it relates to the evolution of functional endoscopic sinus surgery and minimally invasive sinus technique are discussed. The rationale for the authors' departure from Messerklinger's "functional" concepts is also analyzed.

Additionally, endoscopic sinus surgery complications should be distinguished in minor and major based on the treatment they need and the permanent sequelae they can cause. Over the years, the incidence of complications in endoscopic surgery has gone from 8% for the major and 21% for the minor to a percentage of 0 -1.5% and 1.1 – 20.8%, respectively.

Sphenoid sinus is very close to important and vulnerable structures of the skull base and therefore a delayed diagnosis and treatment can be lethal. Thus, the authors provide a review of classification of transsphenoidal skull base approaches and show the main transnasal corridors to the sphenoid sinus based on the anatomical sphenoidal target and extension of pathology.

Lastly, a synopsis of the pathophysiology of post-craniotomy temporomandibular dysfunction and a practical approach to its evaluation and treatment is provided. Several surgical procedures can be used to perform craniotomy, such as the classical pterional, pre-temporal and other fronto-temporal approaches. However, they are all based on the dissection of the temporal muscle, which can lead to a variety of negative side effects.

Chapter 1 - Surgical resection is an optimal curative approach to hepatocarcinoma. When transplantation is not feasible, hepatectomy is the first choice to effectively treat hcc. The 5-year overall survival for the disease stages that benefit from this approach, ranges from 50 to 70%. Unfortunately, only 20-30% of patients are eligible for curative intervention. Moreover, the 5-year-recurrence rate after surgery is close to 70%. Over the last decades, the attempt to reduce recurrence rate, together with a more thorough understanding of the mechanism underlying this phenomenon has lead experts to ask themselves what the best surgical procedure could be. Defining the right extent of the resection is often difficult and unequivocal guidelines have yet to be established. Currently, most international guidelines suggest that the anatomic resection (AR) of a liver segment may allow the removal of the segmental portal bed, preventing microvascular invasion and satellitosis which may be the cause of intrahepatic metastasization (currently ranging between 20 and 70%). Nevertheless, many reports have shown a similar rate of local recurrence (almost 15%) in cases of parenchyma-sparing resection (PSR), where the cancer nodule is removed regardless of the portal segment extension. A recent meta-analysis showed no significant differences in recurrence rate in the two procedures (RR 1.28, 95%CI: 0.59-2.76; p:0.53). No clear advantages can be proven in terms of overall survival, either: the 5-year overall survival rate is 64.9% for AR and 61.1% for PSR. Moreover, PSR was proved to be a safe and oncologically correct technique for cirrhotic patients, for whom preserving as much parenchyma as possible is mandatory to reduce the impact of postoperative liver failure or ascites. In this chapter, the authors will focus on the indications to surgery in hcc, on how to perform a liver resection, and on the different indications to the two main surgical approaches to hepatocellular carcinoma. The authors will discuss long-term outcomes; different theories on the causes of recurrence after resection, and how this evidence could possibly lead to an extension of the indications to a surgical curative approach in primary liver carcinoma.

Chapter 2 - The treatment options for hepatocellular carcinoma (HCC) include liver resection (LR), liver transplantation (LT), transarterial chemoembolization, and local ablation therapy. LR and LT, and local ablation therapy (for small tumors only) provide the best hope for cure. However, most patients with HCC have underlying chronic liver disease (CLD) and are thus at high risk for development of postoperative complications -sometimes fatal- and metachronous multicentric recurrent lesions occurring from the preneoplastic CLD background. Although appropriate treatment is selected for HCC patients with CLD depending on the tumor condition and liver function, a large number of patients are not able to undergo any treatment because of poor liver function and/or complicated tumor condition. This is especially true after repeated treatments for the disease. In the authors' experience of laparoscopic LR (LLR), LLR could expand the indication of LR to severe CLD patients due to its lower damages to the liver and surrounding tissue, especially to collateral circulation around the cirrhotic liver. Child-Pugh score, not class, is one of the promising candidates as a selection indicator which correlates well to the authors' indication criteria of surface small LLR to severe CLD patients, patient's performance status, and prognosis. Portal hypertension should also be counted in the selection criteria. For repeat LLR, there are only small number of reports with small number of patients to date. These studies generally reported that repeat LLR has better short-term outcomes than open (reduced bleedings, less or similar morbidity and shorter hospital stay) without compromising the long-term outcomes. The fact that complete adhesiolysis can be avoided in repeat LLR is also reported. In the comparison of previous procedures, it is reported that the operation time for repeat LLR was shorter for the patients previously treated with LLR than open. Furthermore, it is speculated that LLR for minor repeat LR of cirrhotic liver can be minimized the deterioration of liver function by LR. However, further experience and evaluation of anatomical resection or resections exposing major vessels as repeat LLR, especially after previous anatomical resection, are needed. It is thought that the features of LLR could lead to expanding the indications for LR to those patients in the settings of severe CLD, repeat LR, and bridging to LT. There should be a chance to prolong the overall survival of the patients by using LLR as a powerful local therapy which can be applied repeatedly with minimal deterioration of liver function.

Chapter 3 - Bronchoscopy has become an important procedure, which is performed for diagnostic and therapeutic purposes. There has been very important expansion in the application of bronchoscopy due to technological developments. Bronchoscopic techniques have acquired use as diagnostic procedures in the context of infection or malignancy. Over recent years, procedures such as endobronchial ultrasound have become widely used. Similarly, new technologies such as navigational bronchoscopy are becoming more commonly used. In addition, bronchoscopy has extended its application into interventional procedures.

For example, in the context of Chronic Obstructive Pulmonary Disease, bronchoscopic insertion of endobrochial valves has become widely used. Bronchoscopy also can be used for photodynamic therapy in the context of lung cancer. In this chapter the medical and surgical advances in bronchoscopy will be described.

Chapter 4 - Post-operative pancreatic fistula (POPF) is one of the most dreaded complications in any pancreatic operation given its associated morbidity and mortality. The amylase-rich fluid can cause inflammation, become infected, or cause serious bleeding from neighboring vasculature. POPF are at least as common after distal pancreatectomy than traditional pancreaticoduodenectomy, occurring in approximately 14-30% of all operations. Unlike pancreaticoduodenectomy, there is no pancreatic ductal anastomosis at risk for leakage and disruption; it has been hypothesized that the intact sphincter of Oddi as well as the normal parenchymal texture accounts for the relatively high incidence of POPF following distal pancreatectomy. In a recent meta-analysis, the average rate of clinically relevant POPF was 15.5% with severe POPF requiring reoperation or resulting in organ failure and/or death was 1.3%.

Chapter 5 - Cystic fibrosis (CF) is the most common life threatening autosomal recessive disorder affecting Caucasians. Molecular genetic mutations in the CF transmembrane conductance regulator (CFTR) gene alter function of CFTR protein, which leads to dysfunction in chloride channel on epithelial surface of exocrine glands. In the head and neck area, the pathology involves mostly paranasal sinuses starting from childhood. Chronic and recurrent rhinosinusitis with or without nasal polyposis and mucocele of sinuses are the main disorders observed in CF patients. About 20-25% of these patients will require sinus surgery. Regarding surgical treatment, endoscopic sinus surgery (ESS) for management of paranasal sinus diseases in CF patients is undoubtedly a challenge for the surgeon. Moreover, evidence-based guidelines regarding the precise indications for surgery are currently lacking. Even if ESS is undeniably needed for management of sinonasal complications and can improve CF-related nasal symptoms, its role with regards to timing of surgery and consequent improvement of pulmonary function is not well described. Moreover, underlying medical issues such as acquired coagulopathies and advanced pulmonary disease, raise perioperative morbidity in these patients, with consequent and prolonged hospitalization. Indeed, the surgeon is often faced with distorted anatomy, due to anomalous development of nasal and paranasal structures or multiple revision operations. Therefore, multidisciplinary management of paranasal sinus disease in patients affected by CF is pivotal to achieve the correct surgical indication, prepare the patient for surgery, and address possible perioperative complications. The authors describe the indications of ESS in CF patients, analyzing personal experience in the diagnosis and treatment of CF-related sinus disorders. Finally, data on follow-up after ESS, pulmonary function, and nutritional status will be presented.

Chapter 6 - The minimally invasive sinus technique, (MIST) is different from minimally invasive sinus surgery. MIST implies a treatment philosophy and surgical model that is quite different from functional endoscopic sinus surgery (FESS). The goals of this article are to discuss the origins of functional sinus surgery as it relates to the evolution of FESS and MIST, define MIST as a philosophy and surgical model, discuss treatment of surgical sinus disease, and challenge the rationale for the authors' departure from Messerklinger's "functional" concepts into what will be referred to as "contemporary FESS." Many authors address the reduced revision rate (compared with FESS) following initial intervention with MIST, the potential to markedly reduce the rate of intranasal synechiae, and the reduction in immediate postoperative morbidity.

Chapter 7 - Endoscopic sinus surgery (ESS) is one of the most commonly performed procedures in otolaryngology. ESS complications should be distinguished in minor and major based on the treatment they need and the permanent sequelae they can cause. Over the years it has gone from an incidence of complications in endoscopic surgery of 8% for the major and 21% for the minor to a percentage of 0 -1.5% and 1.1-20.8%, respectively. This is due to the considerable diffusion of the technique with a progressive increase over the years of the surgical experience but their presence help to educate otolaryngologists and patients about complication rates in ESS in a modern context. A complication occurs when injuries to anatomical structures defined in the literature "risk areas" are created. The surgeon must know and identify these areas because these are important land mark that guide the authors' interventions respecting the anatomical boundaries. The aim of this chapter is to describe principle complications and their management.

Chapter 8 - Sphenoid sinus is very close to important and vulnerable structures of the skull base and therefore a delayed diagnosis and treatment can be potentially lethal. Endoscopic sinus surgery is a safe and effective technique that allows a direct route to the sphenoid sinus and therefore is considered the gold standard for the surgical approach to this region. Over the years, the indications for transnasal approaches in skull base surgery have extended in order to obtain an adequate resection of the pathology as with other conventional approaches, with a minor morbidity and an equal efficiency. Many classifications, divided in base of intracranial pathology or intracranial anatomical landmarks, have been proposed to define the transnasal corridors in base of the localization through the middle cranial base. In this chapter, the authors propose a review of classification of transsphenoidal skull base approaches and show the main transnasal corridors to the sphenoid sinus based on the anatomical sphenoidal target and extension of pathology.

Chapter 9 - Chronic rhinosinusitis (CRS) with nasal polyposis (NP) is a common chronic disease that often affects maxillary sinus. Endoscopic sinus surgery (ESS) is the most common procedure to treat the maxillary sinus lesions by a middle meatal antrostomy (MMA) and the introducing of new microdebrider blades of 15, 40, 70, and 120° improved this approach. Nevertheless in some cases, angled microdebrider are not sufficient and canine fossa puncture (CFP) is performed as an alternative method to obtain a complete access to the maxillary antrum.

Chapter 10 - Several surgical procedures can be used to perform craniotomy, such as the classical pterional, pre-temporal and other fronto-temporal approaches. However, they are all based on the dissection of the temporal muscle, which can lead to temporal muscle atrophy, pain in the temporomandibular joint or masticatory muscles, weakness of the jaw closure, and development of signs and symptoms of temporomandibular joint dysfunction, all significantly compromising the patient's quality of life. This type of temporomandibular dysfunction has been frequently neglected as only good results of the primary disease are considered. The following review presents a synopsis of the pathophysiology of post-craniotomy temporomandibular dysfunction and a practical approach to its evaluation and treatment.

In: Handbook of Surgical Procedures
Editor: Heather Gilbert
ISBN: 978-1-53614-580-9

Chapter 1

THE ROLE OF SURGICAL RESECTION IN HEPATOCELLULAR CARCINOMA: ANATOMIC VERSUS PARENCHYMA-SPARING RESECTION AND THEIR ONCOLOGICAL OUTCOMES

Simone Famularo*[*], *MD, Alessandro Giani, MD, Fabio Uggeri, MD, Cristina Ciulli, MD, Luca Nespoli, MD, Giulia Lo Bianco, MD, Luca Arzuffi, MD, Luca Gianotti, MD, ScD and Fabrizio Romano, MD

School of Medicine and Surgery, University of Milan-Bicocca, Italy
Department of Surgery, HPB Unit, San Gerardo Hospital, Monza, Italy

[*] Corresponding Author Email: simone.famularo@gmail.com.

Abstract

Surgical resection is an optimal curative approach to hepatocarcinoma. When transplantation is not feasible, hepatectomy is the first choice to effectively treat hcc. The 5-year overall survival for the disease stages that benefit from this approach, ranges from 50 to 70%. Unfortunately, only 20-30% of patients are eligible for curative intervention. Moreover, the 5-year-recurrence rate after surgery is close to 70%.

Over the last decades, the attempt to reduce recurrence rate, together with a more thorough understanding of the mechanism underlying this phenomenon has lead experts to ask themselves what the best surgical procedure could be. Defining the right extent of the resection is often difficult and unequivocal guidelines have yet to be established. Currently, most international guidelines suggest that the anatomic resection (AR) of a liver segment may allow the removal of the segmental portal bed, preventing microvascular invasion and satellitosis which may be the cause of intrahepatic metastasization (currently ranging between 20 and 70%). Nevertheless, many reports have shown a similar rate of local recurrence (almost 15%) in cases of parenchyma-sparing resection (PSR), where the cancer nodule is removed regardless of the portal segment extension. A recent meta-analysis showed no significant differences in recurrence rate in the two procedures (RR 1.28, 95%CI: 0.59-2.76; p:0.53). No clear advantages can be proven in terms of overall survival, either: the 5-year overall survival rate is 64.9% for AR and 61.1% for PSR. Moreover, PSR was proved to be a safe and oncologically correct technique for cirrhotic patients, for whom preserving as much parenchyma as possible is mandatory to reduce the impact of postoperative liver failure or ascites.

In this chapter, we will focus on the indications to surgery in hcc, on how to perform a liver resection, and on the different indications to the two main surgical approaches to hepatocellular carcinoma. We will discuss long-term outcomes; different theories on the causes of recurrence after resection, and how this evidence could possibly lead to an extension of the indications to a surgical curative approach in primary liver carcinoma.

1. Introduction

Hepatocellular Carcinoma (HCC) is one of the 5 most common malignancies worldwide and the third most common cause of cancer related mortality, accounting for 500,000 deaths globally every year. Although more common in East Asia, the incidence of HCC is constantly increasing in the Western world [1]. Hepatic resection is the first-line therapeutic option and is accepted as a safe treatment, with a proven impact on prognosis and with a low operative mortality, result of the recent innovations in surgical techniques and perioperative management [2]. These advances have improved the outcomes of hepatic resection for HCC, reducing operative morbidity and mortality [3]. However, only 20 to 30% of HCC patients can be candidates to surgical resection because of a poor hepatic reserve function, either caused by underlying chronic liver disease or by HCC multifocal distribution. Although hepatic resection is considered to be a curative treatment for hepatocellular carcinoma, HCC recurrence rate after surgery is quite high, approaching 50% in the first 3 years and reaching 70% in the first 5 years after curative resection [4, 5]. Thus, long term results after surgery remain unsatisfactory. This poor prognosis is commonly alleged to the high incidence of intrahepatic metastasis and of multicentric de novo HCC [6] which develop in accordance with the precancerous status of the remnant diseased liver [7]. With respect to intrahepatic recurrence, macro-portal invasion and intrahepatic metastasis were considered to be the strongest risk factors to affect postoperative prognosis.

However, the role of the different recurrence mechanisms still needs to be clarified. Previously, portal vein dissemination caused by the spreading of HCC cells through the portal vein and its branches was considered the main route for intrahepatic metastasization. This led to the notion that anatomical resection, whose limits are defined by the area of the venous, may prevent intrahepatic metastasization of HCC [8, 9, 10]. Based on this premise, Makuuchi et al. [11] described a correct anatomic resection as the systematic removal of the tumor-bearing hepatic segment confined by its portal tributaries. From a theoretical standpoint, this procedure may be effective in preventing intrahepatic metastasis of HCC. Based on the portal blood flow dissemination theory [12], some authors [13, 14] have used AR for HCC, showing oncological and survival benefits for AR over non-anatomical resections (NAR). However, their results have been debated and no definite conclusion can be drawn from them.

Other authors have reported that AR may prevent hepatic recurrence and prolong survival [15]. In their systematic review of 18 observational studies involving a total of 9036 patients, Cucchetti et al. [12] showed that AR provided a better 5-year overall survival (OS) and disease-free survival (DFS) rate than NAR. Other meta-analyses such as the one by Zhou et al. [16] reported similar results. This data reinforces the theory that AR may reduce the risk of intrahepatic metastasization through portal flow. In a large research project based on Japanese national data analysis, Eguchi et al. [8] also proved a higher RFS rate in AR than in NAR, but a significant statistical difference has not been observed for patients with an HCC larger than 5cm. Despite the advantages shown by these studies, AR can be more difficult to perform and carries more risks than NAR for patients with a low preoperative liver function (e.g., those with cirrhosis). Generally speaking, a larger part of liver parenchyma is resected in AR than in NAR, leading to an increased risk of intraoperative bleeding and to a longer operation time. In clinical practice, surgeons tend to prefer AR when HCC patients display a good liver function, a small-sized tumor, and no cirrhosis.

The evidence of HCC recurrence occurring even in cases treated by hepatic resection and liver transplantation lead to the development of new theories on the pathogenesis of intrahepatic metastasization. According to this new insight, HCC metastatic cells may spread by first migrating through the tumor blood flow (TBF) and then rehoming to the remnant liver [17, 18]. Sakon et al. [19] defined three different patterns of intrahepatic recurrence of HCC as detailed below. Local Intrahepatic Metastasis (IM) (1): HCC recurrence around the tumor by direct spread of the tumor through portal blood flow or venous drainage; Systemic IM (2): HCC recurrence caused by circulating tumor cells (CTCs); MC (3): multicentric HCC recurrence caused by de novo development of HCC. HCC circulating tumor cells have been detected in 81-88% of patients at the time of surgery [20]. Early circulating tumor cells are thought to be spread by portal vein branches [21]. AR aims to resect the liver and the supplying portal vessels respectively in accordance with Couinaud's segments. Thus, theoretically, AR should resect micrometastases (MMTs) within the anatomical segment and reduce the risk of recurrence. It is therefore reasonable to postulate that AR would be more effective than NAR in clearing MMTs and circulating tumor cells, thus decreasing local recurrence (LR) caused by "nearby" MMTs, but not distant recurrence (DR).

Nonanatomic resection (NAR) focuses on achieving a margin-negative liver resection without considering Glisson's pedicle distribution. Because of the high prevalence of underlying liver conditions such as chronic hepatitis and cirrhosis, NAR is often preferred for patients with hepatocellular carcinoma, since it allows sparing of as much liver parenchyma as possible [22]. A cirrhotic liver has a very limited capacity for regeneration and this affects long-term prognosis, which is benefited by parenchyma sparing resections.

Due to the unbalanced distribution of AR and NAR, it was difficult to reach a consensus concerning the advantage of AR in previous studies. Recent studies have failed to confirm the benefits of AR [23, 24] on survival. Okamura et al. and Marubishi et al. [6, 25] have questioned the advantages of AR and showed the incidence of HCC recurrence to be similar on comparing AR and NAR groups. Thus, the effective superiority of AR compared to non-anatomic resection (NAR) remains controversial. Therefore, surgeons must maintain a balance between radical surgery and the need to preserve the function of the remnant liver, which is the focus of the dispute between AR and NAR. No clear advantages could be shown for either of the two techniques in terms of overall survival: the 5-year overall survival rate was 64.9% for AR and 61.1% for PSR. To date, no randomized controlled study has compared outcomes of these two resection methods. The main problem that surgeons face while operating on patients with cirrhosis is balancing the need to achieve a radical intervention while simultaneously preventing the development of postoperative liver failure that could ensue from the removal of too much liver parenchyma. This problem is the basis of the dispute between AR, a theoretically more radical procedure from an oncologic point of view, and

NAR, which reduces the risk of postoperative hepatic failure. The oncological advantage of AR has been actively studied and discussed for decades. The available data is insufficient to prove the prognostic advantage of AR due to the reasons listed below.

First, the definition and surgical technique for AR are not standardized among institutions. Second, the baseline characteristics vary considerably in previous studies making it difficult to determine the pure prognostic advantage of AR, even by meta-analyses, due to the heterogeneity of the target population. Third, because of the significant differences in the preoperative liver function in AR and non-AR populations, a simple prognostic comparison cannot be free from selection bias.

In this chapter we will briefly focus our attention on the surgical indication in HCC, on how to perform a liver resection, and on the different indications to the two main surgical approaches to hepatocellular carcinoma. We will discuss long-term outcomes; the different theories on the mechanisms of recurrence after resection, and show how this evidence could possibly lead to a future extension of the surgical curative approach to primary liver carcinoma.

2. Indication to Surgery

Hepatocellular carcinoma (HCC) is often associated with liver cirrhosis [26]. As a result, the choice of treatment of this pathology is complex and subject to much debate. There is the need to obtain a radical oncological cure, and, at the same time, to ensure the preservation of as much functioning liver parenchyma as possible, considering that it is frequently already compromised by the underlying liver disease. Liver transplantation is theoretically the only possibility for handling both HCC and liver cirrhosis, but this option is not always viable due to the limited availability of organ donors [27]. Moreover, for patients exceeding Milano Criteria, and therefore excluded from transplant, hepatic resection seems the best chance for obtaining a prognostic improvement, reducing morbidity and mortality rates [28].

Nowadays, the most largely accepted algorithm able to direct HCC therapy is based on the Barcelona Clinic Liver Cancer (BCLC) classification (Table 1) developed and validated by the European Association for the Study of Liver Disease (EASL) and by the American Association for the Study of Liver Disease (AASLD) at the end of the last century [29–31] and constantly updated at consensus conferences [32]. In order to determine the patient's prognosis, this classification takes into account preoperative liver status, based on Child-Pugh class, bilirubin levels, presence of portal hypertension, general physical status and local tumor characteristics [33, 34]. It also provides recommendations on therapeutic options, as shown in Table 2. Liver resection, PEI (Percutaneous Ethanol Injection) and thermal ablation with radiofrequency (RFA) are indicated as radical treatments for early-stage tumors. Patients with multiple, large or macrovascular invasive HCC are addressed to palliative treatments, such as TACE (Trans-Arterial Chemo-Embolization), chemotherapy with new agents or others supportive treatments [30].

Table 1. BCLC Classification

Stage	*PST*	*Tumour characteristics*	*Liver functional status*
Stage 0: very early stage HCC	0	Single < 2 cm	No portal hypertension and normal bilirubin
Stage A: early HCC			
A1	0	Single < 5 cm	No portal hypertension and normal bilirubin
A2	0	Single < 5 cm	Portal hypertension and normal bilirubin
A3	0	Single < 5 cm	Portal hypertension and abnormal bilirubin
A4	0	3 tumours < 3 cm	Child-Pugh A-B
Stage B: intermediate HCC	0	Large multinodular (single tumour > 5 cm or 2-3 tumours of which at least one is > 3 cm)	Child-Pugh A-B
Stage C: advanced HCC	1-2	Any tumour with radiological evidence of vascular invasion or extrahepatic spread	Child-Pugh A-B
Stage D: end-stage HCC	3-4	Any	Child-Pugh C

PST: Performance Status Test

In early stage HCC, both surgery and radiofrequency are indicated as first-line treatments, with certain specifications: patients that present multiple comorbidities, elderly patients and, in wider terms, all patients that cannot tolerate a general anesthesia are addressed to radiofrequency. An increased level of bilirubin, portal hypertension or the presence of multiple nodules are also indications to radiofrequency [32]. In selected patients with multinodular HCC, surgical treatment can be associated with intraoperative radiofrequency; this is done, for instance, to achieve radicality on hepatocarcinoma nodules located in anatomically unfavorable positions. Starting from EASL and AASLD recommendations, many local guidelines have been developed by the main liver study groups.

Table 2. Treatment schedule according to BCLC classification

Stage	*Treatment intention*	*First/Second Line treatment*
Stage 0	Radical	Surgical resection
Stage A: early HCC		
A1	Radical	Surgical resection
A2	Radical	Surgical resection → OLT/Percutaneous treatment
A3	Radical	OLT/Percutaneous treatment
A4	Radical	OLT/Percutaneous treatment
Stage B: intermediate HCC	Palliative	Trans-Arterial Chemo-Embolization
Stage C: advanced HCC	Palliative	New agents
Stage D: end-stage HCC	Symptomatic	Supportive treatment

OLT: Orthotopic Liver Transplantation

It is universally accepted that, apart from liver transplantation, and consistently with a BCLC treatment schedule, hepatic resection is the best course of treatment for “very early” or “early” stage HCC. Nevertheless, several single-center reports describe benefits from surgical treatment even for patients with microvascular invasive, multinodular or large HCC. Especially for stage B HCC, the lack of indications to a curative treatment strongly contrasts with clinical practice where, in many centers, patients are addressed to hepatic resection, with a largely demonstrated increase in overall survival (OS) and disease-free survival (DFS) [35–39]. This led to the diffusion of alternative local algorithms, to guide the selection of patients who are eligible to a surgical treatment.

In 2005, Ng et al. demonstrated that even large or multinodular HCC can safely undergo surgical treatment. On a large multi-institutional database of patients treated with hepatic resection in 5 major hepatobiliary centers in Asia, Europe and The United States, they showed a 5-year overall survival of 39% [35]. Ishizawa et al. showed that an adequate patient selection, according to the Child-Pugh class, allows for a dramatic increase in overall survival rates (up to 56%) among Child-Pugh A patients, even in the presence of multiple tumors or portal hypertension [36]. In 2013, Torzilli et al. definitely demonstrated how an update of EASL/AASLD therapeutic guidelines was needed. They conducted a retrospective multicentric survey, showing how, in current clinical practice and in opposition to the existing guidelines, more and more centers recur to surgery for patients with multinodular, large and macrovascular invasive HCC with acceptable short- and long-term results [37]. Almost simultaneously, Bolondi and a panel of experts, proposed a sub-classification of BCLC stage B HCC in order to tailor therapeutic interventions, taking into account the widely emerging data and expert opinions [40, 41]. The staging system was extended as depicted in Table 3.

Taking the lead from this sub-classification, Ciria et al. reported an increase in 5-year overall survival to 62.9%, 28.1% and 15.4%, respectively for B1, B2 and B3-4 stages. They therefore suggested to include this new criteria in the official guidelines [38].

Table 3. BCLC B sub-staging

Sub-stage	*Child-Pugh score*	*Up-to-7 criterion**	*PST*	*PVTT*
B1	5-7	IN	0	NO
B2	5-6	OUT	0	NO
B3	7	OUT	0	NO
B4	8-9	ANY	0-1	NO

* Up-to-7 criterion combines the number of nodules and the major tumour diameter, with the sum being no more than 7.

To our knowledge, the most recent paper on the subject was published in 2018 by Liang et al. It consisted in a systematic review and meta-analysis of Asian data comparing the surgical approach and TACE in intermediate stage HCC. This publication confirmed once again the superiority of hepatic resection in terms of overall survival, without any significant increase in 30-day mortality rates [39]. Given the complexity of the criteria for the surgical approach and their non-universal acceptance, an update in official recommendations is needed. In the meanwhile, a multidisciplinary evaluation of each single case is desirable and useful, in our opinion, since different specialists are potentially involved in the treatment and follow-up of an HCC patient [42].

3. Anatomic Resection (AR) and Parenchyma-Sparing-Resection (PSR)

3.1. Generalities

Recent technical improvements have made hepatectomy for hepatocarcinoma (HCC) an increasingly safe form of curative treatment. However, the long-term survival of patients remains unsatisfactory due to the high rates of recurrence, estimated between 70 and 80% after 5 years [43, 44]. Recurrence can be intrahepatic or multicentric. While different kinds of treatment may suppress liver fibrosis and thus prevent multicentric recurrence, intrahepatic recurrence seems to be closely related to local vascular invasion, thus making anatomical resection (AR) the best technique to prevent it, from a theoretical standpoint [45].

Microportal invasion and intrahepatic metastasis were once considered to be the most important factors leading to recurrence and were associated with poor prognosis [46, 47]. On this basis, Makuuchi et al. first described AR in 1985 [48]. The procedure is based on the systematic removal of a liver segment with its tributary portal branches and should theoretically allow the elimination of intrahepatic micro metastasis improving patient survival. The long-term outcome after resection of hepatocellular carcinoma, however, is also influenced by factors related to the characteristics of the tumor and by the underlying liver disease.

Today the choice between anatomical resection (AR) and non anatomical (NAR) resection for HCC is controversial. From an oncological point of view, AR appears to be superior to NAR, enabling to obtain negative margins and leading to a better 2-year recurrence rate for high grade aggressive tumors, as it permits the removal of satellite lesions and microvascular invasion [23]. Moreover, the better control of the vascular pedicle in AR allows for a reduced intraoperative blood loss, leading to a lower rate of postoperative morbidity and mortality [49]. In fact, NAR results in a higher incidence of biliary fistula and infection because of the higher percentage of remnant devitalized liver tissue [7]. To understand the vascular and biliary anatomy of the liver is mandatory for a successful AR. Since HCC usually develops over a background of liver cirrhosis, it is important that anatomical resection be able to clear the tumor and still leave a sufficient amount of liver to avoid postoperative liver failure.

The concept of anatomical resection is based on the division of the liver into segments first described by Healy in 1953 [50] and updated by Couinaud in 1957 [51]. Nowadays, from a surgical-functional point of view, we no longer divide the liver into lobes, according to classic topographic anatomy, but, more correctly, into segments based on portal, arterial and biliary branching. The liver, as proposed by Couinaud [51], is therefore divided into four sectors, each delimited by a branch of the portal vein; sectors are further divided into segments for a total of eight, conventionally indicated with the corresponding Roman number. The projection, on the upper surface of the liver, of the course of the mean hepatic vein (the main portal fissure, corresponds to the ideal line connecting the left margin of the cava vein to the bottom of the gallbladder) divides the organ into two hemi-livers: right and left, provided with an autonomous vascular and biliary supply. The two hemi-livers are in turn divided into two sectors from the left and right portal fissures (Figure 1). The right portal fissure corresponds to the course of the right hepatic vein and is projected on an ideal line that from the right margin of the vena cava points anteriorly to the middle point between the right margin of the liver and the right margin of the gallbladder (Figure 1). The left portal fissure corresponds to the course of the left hepatic vein and is projected on an ideal line that from the left margin of the vena cava reaches the left margin of the liver (Figure 1). Starting from the right lobe of the liver and moving towards the left, you can distinguish:

- The *right lateral sector*: formed by the VII° (above) and VI° segment (below)
- The m*edial right sector*: formed by the VIII ° (above) and V° segment (below)
- The l*eft medial sector:* formed by the I° and IV° segments (lateral) and by the IV° and III ° segments (medial)
- The l*eft lateral sector*: formed by the II° segment (Figure 2)

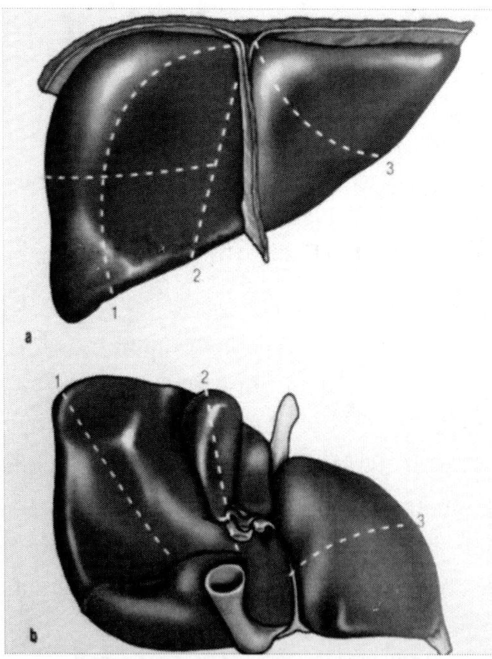

Figure 1. Representation on the anterior (a) and inferior (b) surface of the liver, of the portal fissures and of the division in segments: 1) right portal fissure; 2) main or median portal fissure; 3) right portal fissure.

The scientific committee of the International Hepato-Pancreato-Biliary Association proposed the Brisbane 2000 Terminology of Liver Anatomy and resection [52] to define a universal terminology with which to refer to liver anatomy. According to this terminology, first the liver is divided into two parts, the main liver and the caudate lobe (called I° segment by Couinaud). Then the main liver is divided into the right and left liver. The practical applications of this subdivision is proven by the fact that this terminology has gained wide acceptance removing most of the confusion that existed in the past.

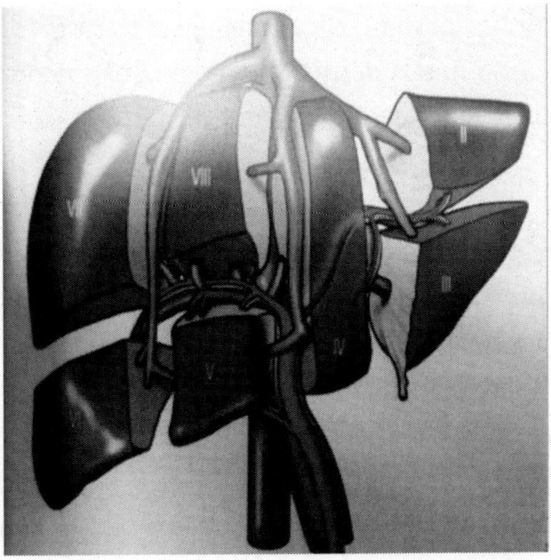

Figure 2. Subdivision of the liver into segments according to Couinaud.

To perform a precise anatomical liver dissection it is necessary to accurately identify the segments and the portal fissures during resection. Different methods of segment identification are employed both in conventional hepatic surgery and in laparoscopy. The most widely tested methods are the tattooing method [48, 53] and the Glissonian approach [54, 55], which is especially simple to perform. Other techniques have been experimented; some Authors inject intravenous indocyanine green after clamping the Glissonian pedicle to better define the resection margins [56]. The aim of this section is to describe the various techniques currently used to perform an anatomical resection of the liver in the presence of HCC.

3.2. Anatomical Resection

As already described, anatomical resection refers to the resection of the tumor-involved segment or section, together with its portal vein branch, resected *en bloc*. This approach includes: left or right hepatectomy, hemihepatectomy, segmentectomy and subsegmentectomy, sectionectomy and trisectionectomy, based on Couinaud's classification. In sectionectomy, the resection line is defined by a demarcation on the liver surface after ligation of the sectional pedicle and of the trunk of the hepatic vein exposed on the resected surface [42].

3.2.1. Glissonian Approach

The approach to the Glissonean pedicle has enabled us to obtain new knowledge of liver anatomy which lead to an improvement of surgical techniques. This approach starts with an extra fascial access to the hepatic hilum. The secondary Glissonean pedicles are taped and ligated at the hepatic hilum without parenchyma dissection. Dissection starts above the hilar plate so that the surgeon does not have to take into account possible artery and bile duct anatomic variations. Tertiary branches can be approached through the hepatic hilum or through the liver parenchyma at the margin between segments [57]. The Glisson capsule is made up of connective tissue covering the peduncle, which in turn contains the hepatic artery, portal vein and bile duct. The Glisson capsule is connected to the liver capsule and to the hepatoduodenal ligament forming a thick plate on the inferior face of the liver, which is referred to as the "hilar plate."

The first dissection of the hepatoduodenal ligament elements during hepatectomy was performed around 1950 and the procedure was defined as the first hepatectomy with controlled method [58]. By contrast, a few years later, other Authors started dissecting the liver parenchyma, approaching and ligating the portal pedicles intra-hepatically [59, 60]. These two approaches are recognized as being the basic techniques for anatomic liver resection [61]. Couinaud et al. [62] and Takasaki et al. [54] first reported the Glissonian approach to the hepatic hilus respectively in 1985 and 1986. Couinaud [63] later described three different ways to approach Glissonean pedicles: *the intrafascial, the extrafascial,* and *the extrafascial and transfissural approaches.*

The *intrafascial approach* involves a conventional dissection of the hepatoduodenal ligament. Dissection is performed below the hilar plate, making the procedure unsafe, and surgeons have to take into account possible anatomic variations of the hepatic artery and bile ducts. In the *extra-fascial approach,* instead, the pedicle is dissected first through the hepatic parenchyma and then extra-hepatically at the hilum. In the *extra-fascial and transfissural approach* the main portal fissure or left supra-hepatic fissure are opened after dissecting the liver parenchyma, and surgeons can therefore appreciatc the direction and distribution of the pedicles that arise from the hilar plate. This procedure involves major hepatic transections along the main portal branches or the umbilical fissure [59, 60]. The extrafascial approach is further separated into the *intrahepatic* and *extrahepatic* approaches depending on the presence or absence of parenchymal destruction. Intrahepatic isolation can possibly lead to unexpected injury of the portal pedicle or hepatic vein, therefore extrahepatic Glissonean pedicle isolation should be considered the ideal procedure [64].

To approach the right Glissonean pedicle the procedure provides that, after cholecystectomy, the cystic plate be dissected. Behind the cystic plate, the right anterior Glissonian pedicle can then be recognized and approached carefully after having detached the hilar plate from the liver parenchyma. Subsequently, the pedicle is completely dissected and clamped to confirm the extension of the area supplemented by its flow. The right, posterior pedicle can then be taped after the main pedicle is. Afterwards, the tape is pulled at the ramification between the anterior and right posterior pedicle. This procedure allows us to evidence the area of altered parenchymal staining after clamping and the site of the neoplasm as confirmed by ultrasound. At this point the pedicle must be ligated and dissected before going further with the liver section [55].

The approach to the left pedicle was first described by Couinaud in 1985 [62]. Dissection starts to the left of the hilus and is then conducted along the ventral surface of the Arantius duct. Finally the pedicle is encircled and clamped. Some liver surgeons have attempted to reproduce these methods in laparoscopy, but, due to the anatomic complexity of the liver and to the inherent limitations of the laparoscopic technique, this has proven difficult. The recent introduction of robotic techniques has enhanced the possibilities of performing minimally invasive liver surgical procedures. Recently, Lee et al. [65] reported a series of 10 patients subjected to an extrahepatic right approach of the Glissonean pedicle by robotic route. Four robotic ports and one assistant port were used. The falciform and ipsilateral coronary ligament were sectioned, the inferior and posterior sides of the liver freed from the diaphragm and the plane of the inferior vena cava exposed. The liberation of the right liver is achieved through the section of accessory hepatic veins. The selected Glissonean pedicle is then dissected by the extrafascial approach, at the hepatic hilus for the right resections and at the level of the round ligament for medial and lateral sectionectomy.

When resection is first conducted along the right or left side of the round ligament, parenchymal transection is performed to expose Glissonian pedicles. In right posterior sectionectomy, the gallbladder is retracted upwards to expose the hepatic hilus and the portal branches that supply the I° segment, which are sectioned to expose the main portal branches. Once the pedicle has been identified, it is encircled and closed with a laparoscopic clamp. Clamping produces an ischemic demarcation on the line of hepatic transection that is then marked with an electrocautery hook. Finally, an intraoperative ultrasound examination is performed to confirm the location of the neoplasm and the extension of surgical margins.

3.2.2. Indocyanine Green

In hepatobiliary surgery, the fluorescence and bile excretion of indocyanine green (ICG) can be used for real-time visualization of biological structures. Intra-operatory fluorescence imaging can be used to identify subcapsular hepatic tumors and to define the limits of hepatic segments. The limits of hepatic segments can be visualized through the injection of ICG in the portal vein or after intravenous injection following the closure of the portal pedicle proximal to the region that has to be removed. This technique enables the identification of liver segments before surgical resection and during parenchymal transection for anatomic resections. Intraoperative fluorescence imaging is able to localize the neoplastic lesion thanks to the biliary secretion disorders that are characteristic of the neoplastic tissue of hepatocellular carcinoma and of the hepatic parenchyma surrounding adenocarcinoma [66].

Fluorescence imaging following portal injection of IGC was used for the first time in 2008 for the identification of hepatic segments [67]. Since then, the technique has been improved by combining a more diluted ICG solution (2.5 mg) to an imaging system able to merge fluorescence images with color images [68]. The concomitant injection of indigo-carmine solution (an organic salt derived from indigo by sulfonation) and IGC can increase the rate of identification of the liver segments, especially in patients affected with cirrhosis or that have undergone previous surgery, where the presence of connective tissue can mask the hepatic surface [69].

In addition to identifying hepatic segments after portal injection of ICG (*positive staining technique*), hepatic segments can also be identified as ischemic areas through intravenous injection of ICG after closure of the corresponding portal pedicle (*negative staining technique*) [68, 70]. Intraoperative fluorescence imaging may also allow us to estimate portal uptake in veno-occlusive regions of the liver during hepatectomy [71].

The use of indocyanine green in localizing the neoplastic lesion in need for removal is also useful in minimally invasive surgery, where the possibilities of inspection and manipulation are limited compared to open surgery. Furthermore, the negative staining technique is particularly useful in laparoscopy where injection of ICG into the portal vein is technically difficult [70, 72]. When the V° VI° VII° VIII° liver segments have to be approached, different difficulties may arise that make it harder to perform the operation in laparoscopy, while intraoperative ultrasound may be difficult due to the impossibility of freely handing the ultrasound probe.

In this regard, Ueno et al. [56] reported a new technique for liver segment identification in laparoscopic surgery. They previously performed a laparoscopic splenectomy concomitant with interventional radiology for hypersplenism to reduce intraoperative blood loss. With this technique the authors tried to overcome the difficulty of dye injection during laparoscopic intraoperative ultrasound. At first they mobilized the liver, then, from the right femoral artery, they inserted a 3 French (Fr) sheath catheter, under the guide of preoperative simulation images. Two other catheters of 3 and 1.9 Fr respectively were inserted into the celiac artery and into the targeted arterial branches. After confirming the perfusion area through arteriography, a mixed dye solution including ICG was injected into the target and the branches were embolized using gelatin particles.

The mixed dye solution was composed of: 2 mL of a diluted IGC solution, 2 mL of indigo carmine water, 1 mL of Sonazoid solution and 1 mL of a contrast medium. As an embolic agent 1 mm of porous gelatin particles were mixed with 3 mL of a mixed dye solution and 10 mL of a contrast medium. At this point about 3 ml of mixed dye solution were slowly injected into the target and the targeted branches were then embolized. When performed under fluoroscopy monitoring, this technique requires a hybrid operating room. Immediately after the injection of the dye solution mixture, visual alterations can be observed on the surface of the liver, along with ICG fluorescent margins, that define the intraparenchymal cutting line.

3.3. Parenchyma Sparing Liver Resection

Liver resection often represents the treatment of choice for both primary and secondary liver malignancies [73]. Depending on tumor location, dimension and diffusion major resections may be required to achieve an adequate oncologic result. Volume of remnant liver is crucial to avoid postoperative liver failure, especially in cirrhotic patients or in patients submitted to neoadjuvant chemotherapy. In order to reduce the substantial morbidity and mortality associated with major liver resections, attention has focused on the technical possibility of sparing as much liver as possible while aiming at achieving, at the same time, an effective oncological result.

A better knowledge of tumor biology and of its influence on local recurrence and survival, and the development of intraoperative ultrasound skills, constitute the basis of the so-called "parenchymal sparing liver surgery." The term parenchymal sparing resection (PSR) encompasses a wide range of resections, ranging from non anatomical, small, wedge resection to more complex non-anatomical atypical resections.

3.3.1. Preoperative and Intraoperative Planning

The prerequisite for PSR is a careful and meticulous evaluation of the relationship between hepatic lesions of hepatic veins and the glissonian pedicles. This evaluation allows the planning of the ideal anatomical roadmap for a proper resection, preserving an adequate blood inflow and outflow from the spared parenchyma. CT scanning and MRI are usually employed preoperatively for this purpose and give the possibility for different image reconstruction techniques, including 3D imaging [74, 75]. Although displaying a suboptimal sensitivity for smaller (<1 cm) lesions, triphasic CT scanning allows us to obtain an optimal vascular and lesion assessment. Moreover, it allows for concomitant volumetric assessment of the remnant liver [76].

MRI, with the use of liver-specific contrast agents, offers a good sensitivity for smaller hepatic nodules also. Moreover, it provides a good visualization of the biliary tree anatomy, useful for planning an ideal resection plane. Intraoperative imaging through ultrasound (IOUS) is essential in PSR, since it allows the localization of even small or deep-located nodules and "navigation" into the liver following the planned resection plane precisely, visualizing and preserving vascular and biliary structures [77]. IOUS allows for a complete investigation of the vascular anatomy of the liver: hepatic veins and accessory hepatic veins can be visualized, as well as the presence of communicating vessels within adjacent hepatic veins. These communicating vessels allow us to perform a PSR even in the presence of a neoplastic involvement of a hepatic vein at a hepatic-caval confluence. They preserve an adequate venous outflow from the spared parenchyma. A successful PSR, especially in complex cases, requires excellent expertise in using this technique, as well as high quality equipment.

3.3.2. Surgical Techniques

The definition of PSR encompasses different kinds of liver resection able to maximize the liver remnant volume if compared with other, more extended, techniques.

4. Long Term Outcomes and Risk Factors

One of the best curative approaches for hepatocellular cancer is liver resection [78]. This procedure is the first choice of treatment when transplantation is not feasible. Hepatic resection for HCC is safe and now displays a low operative mortality due to an improvement in pre-operative management, surgical technique and postoperative care [2]. The most important concern is the high rate of postoperative recurrence of HCC. This situation affects about 50%-60% of patients during the first 3 years and 70-90% during the first 5 years after curative hepatectomy [79, 80]. During the last decades, authors have tried to understand the pathological mechanism of HCC metastasization and the best surgical approach to reduce the recurrence rate of this tumor. Some authors underline that microscopic vascular invasion and peripheral spread of the primary tumor could cause subclinical metastases and that these could be the most important factors affecting the long term prognosis of these patients [46, 81]. Based on this premise, an extensive resection should be the best treatment for HCC. On the other hand, a massive resection can be difficult to operate on a damaged liver. HCCs frequently arise in cirrhosis. The cirrhotic liver has a limited capacity for regeneration [82]. In these cases a limited resection is mandatory, since another important cause of mortality after hepatic resection is liver failure. A limited resection could improve long term survival allowing us to preserve hepatic function and leave room for other therapeutic options [83]. The most widespread methods for patients undergoing liver resection for HCC are anatomic resection (AR) and non anatomic resection (NAR) [12, 16]. There is limited evidence supporting one of these techniques over the other [7, 84]. Several studies have compared these two techniques but they do not clearly show the advantages of AR over NAR. There are studies showing that AR improves overall survival and disease free survival since it allows for a complete removal of tumor bearing portal tributaries [83, 85–88]. Other evidence shows no advantages of AR when compared to NAR [25, 45, 89]. AR is often indicated in patients with low-degree liver damage, while NAR is usually considered the best approach when preserving liver parenchyma and function is mandatory. The best treatment must balance resectability and preservation of liver function. The conclusion of this debate is very difficult due to the heterogeneity of studies and to the absence of randomized controlled trials. Long term outcomes can be evaluated in terms of overall survival (OS), disease free survival (DFS) and local recurrence (LR). In their study, Yamamoto et al. described a 1- and 2-year OS rate of 92.1% and 85.8% for AR and NAR, respectively, and DFS rates of 78.2% and 63%. These data suggest that there is no significant difference in terms of OS and DFS between the two groups. Furthermore, a longer hospital stay and a greater blood loss was found during surgery in the AR group. A better DFS was found in some AR subgroups. For example AR was better than NAR for patients with a tumor size of 2-5 cm suggesting that there is no difference in surgical technique when tumor size is less than 2 cm [90]. This finding could be referred to a higher tendency of larger HCCs to form intrahepatic or other organ metastasis. In the HCV positive subgroup, authors found a better DFS in the AR group. This group of patients could benefit from AR since HCV patients have a higher rate of intrahepatic metastasis compared to HBV positive patients [91]. Cucchetti et al. compared AR and NAR in Child A patients. In this study, the authors stratified the population according to time to recurrence (early vs late), tumor diameter and tumor differentiation, finding no difference between

NAR and AR. AR is better than NAR when tumor diameter is larger, when there is microvascular invasion, in G3-G4 degrees and in early recurrence. On the contrary, for small, G1-G2 degree tumors, AR loses its superiority. Another important finding is that there is no difference in the rate of late recurrence in the two groups.

The rationale is to approach the patients through AR when the tumor is larger, in the presence of microvascular invasion or when the tumor is poorly differentiated. NAR is recommended when liver functionally is low or when there are no unfavorable tumor features [86]. These features can be identified during preoperative workup. Some authors related tumor size to tumor differentiation and to the presence or absence of microvascular invasion. Others identified tumor size, number, and Edmondson grade as microvascular invasion predictors. These data could be useful for surgical decision making [92, 93]. Tanaka et al. compared AR to NAR in 125 patients undergoing hepatic resection for HCC. In this study, the 1-, 3- and 5-year hepatic recurrence rates were found to be 20%, 53% and 64% in AR as opposed to 21%, 52% and 76% in NAR. The 1-, 3- and 5- year OS were respectively 96%, 70% and 54% in AR and 97%, 91% and 61% in NAR. This study showed no significant difference between anatomic and non anatomic liver resection.

At a univariate and multivariate analysis, type of resection was found not to affect survival. Furthermore, AR and NAR showed no difference in number and site of recurrent locations. In this study, authors also studied patients undergoing a second liver resection for recurrence. In patients with liver cirrhosis, the tax of second resections was higher in the non-anatomic resection group. Anyway, the proportion of patients surviving after recurrence was 16% in AR as opposed to 36% in NAR. This data probably depends on a better preservation of liver parenchyma in non anatomic resection compared to anatomic resection.

In the end, looking at patients in which a recurrence with three or more nodules has occurred, no differences were found in AR groups compared to NAR groups. Moreover, no patient had a recurrence at the margins of the resection [23].

Marubashi et al. studied recurrence patterns after NAR and AR. In this study they observed substantial differences between the two groups. Liver function of patients in the NAR group was worse than in the AR group. ICG15R, Child-Pugh score, and degree of live damage were also better in AR patients. On the contrary, AR groups included patients with a larger tumor size, higher serum tumor markers and a higher tax of microvascular invasion.

Univariate and multivariate analysis have shown that the type of liver resection was not a risk factor for tumor recurrence. This study underlined that serum AST, tumor size, multiplicity, serum albumin level and estimated blood loss were independent risk factors for HCC recurrence. Authors evaluated three different aspects of HCC recurrence: area of HCC recurrence, number of recurrent tumors and location of the recurrence. Comparing HCC recurrence patterns no difference could be detected between the two different groups. Only 1.4% of patients had a local recurrence, in the other cases recurrence was the result of systemic dissemination or de novo development. This study confirmed that the type of surgical resection to HCC is not a risk factor of recurrence. It also confirmed how the selection of the surgical method should be based on the clinical status of the patient [94]. These studies underline that the type of surgical resection is not a risk factor for HCC recurrence and consequently, does not affect long term outcomes. These results suggest there are others factor that influence prognosis more than the type of surgery.

Some studies report that HCV infection, Child-Pugh class B, AST $\geq$ 35 UI/L, PLT <14 X 10^4 microliter, ICG-R15 $\geq$25%, AFP $\geq$20 ng/mL, cancer spread and cirrhosis affect DFS. Child-Pugh class B, PLT <14 X 10^4 microliter, ICG-R15 $\geq$25%, AFP $\geq$20 ng/mL, cancer spread, cirrhosis and infiltration into the capsule seem to affect OS, instead [45]. Another study found that preoperative serum AST, prothrombin time, tumor size, albumin, multiplicity and estimated blood loss were independent risk factors for HCC recurrence. This study further demonstrated that the resection method does not affect HCC recurrence [94]. These data suggest that the clinical status influences long-term prognosis more than the kind of liver resection.

Tomimaru et al. studied retrospectively a selected population affected by HCC. Authors selected a population with a small solitary HCC (≤ 3cm) without macroscopic vascular invasion and with an adequate underling liver function. This study showed no differences in short-term and long-term outcomes. Furthermore, univariate analysis proved that the presence of HBV, HCV, microscopic invasion and number of microscopic tumors affect DFS. HCV and microscopic vascular invasion were linked to DFS in multivariate analysis as well. On the other hand, the number of microscopic tumors, HCV and liver cirrhosis were related to OS at univariate analysis, while only the number of microscopic tumors was connected to OS at multivariate analysis [95]. These results underline the importance of the patients' clinical background and of tumor features. The presence of a chronic inflammation of the liver, cirrhosis, the presence of microvascular inflammation or multiple nodules are risk factors for recurrence and affect short-term and long-term outcomes.

Eguchi et al. compared AR and NAR in a cohort of 5781 patients with a single HCC. Stratifying patients for tumor size, they found that HCCs ranging from 2 cm to 5 cm benefit from AR rather than NAR. Furthermore, in HCCs smaller than 2 cm, no difference was found in long-term survival. Authors also stratified patients for liver function. In this respect, differences between AR and NAR disappeared, also, for tumors larger than 2 cm [84]. Our group tried to compare long term outcomes of NAR and AR. In this study we used a propensity score analysis to reduce biases. We analyzed retrospectively 455 patients. We found an OS of 47.6 months for AR and 56.5 months for NAR ($p= 0.169$). The median DFS was 29.2 months for AR and 24.9 months for NAR ($p=0.337$). At univariate analysis, we found that the presence of cirrhosis, BCLC stage, microvascular invasion, satellitosis, surgical resection margins, postoperative liver failure, postoperative ascites, number of nodules, size of nodules and ALBI grade were associated with a reduction in OS. Using a multivariate regression model, we found that cirrhosis, microvascular invasion, BCLC grade B, presence of satellitosis, postoperative ascites, grade 3-4 Clavien-Dindo classification and ALBI grade 2 were independently associated with OS. Furthermore, cirrhosis, BCLC grade, microvascular invasion, presence of satellitosis, postoperative ascites and number of nodules were all associated with early recurrence (DFS < 2 years). At the multivariate Cox regression model: presence of cirrhosis, grade B BCLC, microvascular invasion and satellitosis were independently associated with the risk of recurrence.

Our study demonstrated no differences between AR and NAR as well. Furthermore, we also appreciated the importance of liver function and tumor characteristics as the most important factors affecting OS and DFS. In the end, studies suggested that the type of surgery is not an independent risk factor for HCC recurrence. Tumor-related factors appear to be more relevant than type of surgery in affecting the risk of HCC recurrence.

5. Recurrence Pattern after Resection: Intra-Hepatic Metastasis or De-Novo Recurrence

Pattern of recurrence is a main topic in HCC therapeutic strategies. The peculiarity of this tumor is the background parenchyma in which it develops. In the majority of cases it is characterized by a chronic inflammatory state rather than by outright cirrhosis. In fact, when a new nodule is diagnosed, or when the tumor arises as a multinodular disease, no clinical or biochemical features are able to distinguish between the occurrence of a de-novo nodule (multicentric occurrence, MO), favoured by the chronic underlying inflammatory state of the liver, and the real intrahepatic metastasization (IM) of a primitive lesion. The ability to distinguish between these two occurrences would affect our interpretation of the phenomenon and change the current figures on hepatocarcinoma recurrence.

These considerations become fundamental when we consider that multinodular disease currently has no indication to curative treatment although it could possibly be the expression of de-novo multicentric carcinogenesis rather than of intrahepatic metastasization. The effect of cirrhosis on recurrence has been recently investigated by Sasaki et al. [96], who compared cirrhotic and healthy patients. Their results showed how cirrhosis can affect the pattern of recurrence, increasing the chances of MO [19] over IM.

However, they reported a comparable rate of early recurrence, which they interpreted as the expression of the metastatic potential intrinsic in hepatocellular carcinoma. Thus, a cirrhotic liver, when compared to a healthy one, seems to be characterized by the possibility of metastasization, as well as by the occurrence of de-novo neoplasm through the chronic inflammatory boost of the underlying cirrhosis. In the last decade, experimental genetic analysis has allowed us to improve our knowledge of recurrence patterns in HCC. Studies on Asian databases described an IM rate of between 50-70% after liver surgery [97–99]. The same authors reported how the IM pattern seems to have a worse prognosis compared to tumors that recur with a MO pattern [98–100]. A recent meta-analysis has confirmed this trend on seven reports [100], all of them on Asiatic data. To the best of our knowledge, no western data is available in literature regarding the incidence of the two patterns. Many efforts have been made to understand the different conditions that lead to IM rather than MO. Most studies point out the main role of the MVI as "primum-movers" in the metastasization pathway [101–103].

The role of microvascular invasion in recurrence was first explored by Makuuchi et al. in 1985 [48]. The authors reported a rate of 73% of 62 HCC patients showing a microscopic tumor thrombus in the portal venous branch. From this manuscript came the proposal of a resection technique able to cut off the tumour portal supply according to Coinaud segmentation. This approach should allow the reduction of the rate of recurrence. Up to now, there is still no accord among the multiple experiences all over the world concerning the real impact of this approach on recurrence. According to a recent systematic review, the rate of microscopic portal vein thrombosis in the tumor area is definitely smaller than expected, varying according to different tumor sizes: 0.5% for early cancer, 16.2% for tumors of less than 2 cm, 17.4% when size is <5cm, as high as 64% for tumors larger than 5 cm [104]. Furthermore, the theory of cancer spread through portal circulation is not able to explain the rate of recurrence after transplantation, a very rare but possible occurrence.

Over the last few years, especially through the Osaka Hospital (Japan) experience, new data has emerged that could clarify the mechanism of intrahepatic metastasization. CT studies during arterial portography and hepatic arteriography allowed Sakon et al. to define three different patterns of intrahepatic recurrence. 1) Local IM: HCC recurrence around the tumor, caused by direct spread through the portal blood flow or venous drainage; 2) Systemic IM: HCC recurrence caused by circulating tumor cells; 3) MC: multicentric HCC recurrence caused by de-novo development of hepatocarcinoma [17–19, 104]. These authors also evidenced the role of tumor blood flow (TBF) drainage, which appears at CT scan as the vascular supply area of the tumor, which is not always directly related to the segmental portal branch distribution around the nodule. They stated how the different patterns of recurrence are significantly associated with different TBF drainage patterns.

Local diffusion is the manifestation of anatomical dissemination (depicted by the portal vein type at TBF drainage) rather than non-anatomical (represented by the marginal or hypovascular TBF type). More recently, Marubashi et al. underlined the importance of overcoming the old theory of portal vein dissemination as the main route for intrahepatic metastasization, favoring the tumor blood flow drainage theory over the systemic rehoming theory [6].

Given the different types of recurrence that can occur in the context of hepatocarcinoma, there are still few reports about the real impact of surgery on reducing recurrence rate. As already discussed, most physicians assume that, when metastasization is due to MVI, a radical excision of the anatomical liver segment with its portal vascularization, should achieve the best outcome in terms of recurrence [10, 105, 106]. However, many authors have reported no differences between AR and PSR in long term-oncological outcomes [107, 108]. A recent, combined Asian and Western-based study [109] showed no differences in long-term outcomes between the two surgical techniques. AR seems to reduce the rate of early recurrence in cancers with MVI or with a G3-4 differentiation pattern according to Edmonson's histological classification. Early recurrence has been defined as a possible clinical indicator of the metastasization pattern in HCC [100, 101, 109]. Marubashi et al. [6] compared the two surgical techniques and their respective patterns of recurrence. No significant differences were evident in the local dissemination rate after surgery, neither when comparing intrahepatic and extrahepatic recurrences, nor on the localization of the recurrent nodules. These results reflect the difficulty in estimating the real impact of different recurrence patterns on long terms outcomes.

Lesions characterized by a different tumor burden can express different carcinogenic potentials. This power is independent of the surgical technique. In fact, according to the "re-homing theory" [17, 18], used to explain recurrence after transplantation, once the hepatocellular nodule acquires the features of invasiveness, metastasization can equally occurin the liver and in the blood flow, so that neither of the currently available therapies can possibly reduce or cancel the risk of recurrence.

Others studies, analyzing recurrence patterns after surgical resection, presented similar results. Local dissemination after PSR apparently concerns just a minority of cases, most HCC recurrences being apparently caused by systemic dissemination of circulating tumor cells or multicentric occurrence of de-novo HCC [6, 22]. According to these considerations, it may be easy to understand the importance of finding a procedure able to distinguish between IM and MO.

Different efforts have been made to distinguish the two patterns by genetic analyses. CGH-arrays, microsatellite instability, loss of heterozygosity and other genetic features have been diffusely employed to characterize the differences between a primitive nodule and its recurrence. More recently, variations of the mitochondrial DNA of hepatocellular carcinoma were explored, with interesting results and good sensitivity and specificity [110]. These procedures, however, are affected by the impossibility of predicting a recurrence pattern during the preoperative work-up.

Genetic analysis can only be performed on histological specimens, so that the real nature of the treated lesion can only be recognized aposteriori. Shimada et al. [111] reported C hepatitis infection, a platelet count of<10x10^4/microl; tumor size and histological gradeas independent factors in differentiating MO from IM. Nakano et al. [111, 112] reported that a tumor capsule was rarely observed in IM patients. Different authors stated that large and multinodular HCC have always presented a high incidence of recurrence, and that these types of multinodular HCCs were more usually identified as IM [113, 114]. More recently, a recurrence-free interval of over 18 months after initial hepatic resection has been suggested as a cut-off point to differentiate MO from IM in clinical practice [115]. Other authors have pointed out a cut-off of 2 years for RFS [116].

However, some retrospective series do not support this clinical approach, recording no difference in outcomes when time to recurrence is employed to distinguish between different recurrent patterns and to predict different outcomes of AR and PSR. Until now, no reliable and universally accepted clinical models are available to predict the pattern of recurrence of HCC. To conclude, PSR seems comparable to AR as a treatment for hepatic cancer. Where recurrence is concerned, distant intrahepatic recurrence is more common than surgical hedge relapse or distant metastases. This evidence further points towards the need for a reinterpretation of the mechanism underlying recurrence in hepatocarcinoma, revisiting the portal-flow-theory and our general approach to the disease.

6. Extending the Role of Surgery: From Benchmark to Bedside

To better address these clinical questions, molecular characterization has been performed on multiple liver tumor specimens through various analyses, using new biological mechanisms and molecular markers. In recent years, a better knowledge of mutational and epigenetic events deregulating the signaling pathways involved in tumor progression, and the definition of different genetic variants of HCC, have allowed a better of recurrence patterns, the prediction of disease outcomes and the identification of potential prognostic markers and targets for molecular-based personalized therapies [117, 118]. Some studies used the HBV-DNA integration pattern, the X chromosome inactivation assay, and comparative genomic hybridization (CGH) as possible markers of tumor clone origin [119, 120]. However, all of these methods have inherent limitations. They can be applied only to HCC patients with integrated HBV-DNA, only to female patients or require expensive equipment and reagents, respectively.

Moreover, HBV integration testing through southern blotting requires a consistent amount of DNA genome [121]. Micro-satellite polymorphism, including loss of heterozygosity (LOH) and microsatellite instability (MSI) are important genetic features in carcinogenesis. LOH analysis of specific DNA microsatellite loci were performed in the attempt to distinguish IM of monoclonal origin, from multiclonal MO [98, 122]. Compared to other molecular methods, the test of microsatellite polymorphism with Polymerase Chain Reaction (PCR) and Polyacrylamide Gel Electrophoresis (PAGE) shows many advantages. Moreover, it can be used on small quantities of DNA genome that can be acquired from tiny specimens such as fine-needle biopsy specimens. DNA microarray technology is currently employed in identifying specific gene expression signatures of HCC. Recently, this technique has been used to predict early HCC recurrence due to intrahepatic metastasis; however, no well-defined predictors for late recurrence have been discovered. Some studies have focused on the characteristics of non-tumorous liver to predict late recurrence due to de novo hepatocarcinogenesis. These studies were based on the idea of "field cancerization" but did not lead to conclusive results [123]. In another study [124], the gene expression signature of primary metastatic HCCs was found to be similar to that of the corresponding IMs, implying that the genetic deregulation responsible for metastasization initiates within the primary tumor. The Adrenomedullin (AM) gene was identified as a leader gene overexpressed in HCCs with IM, while a different gene expression profile was observed in multicentric HCCs [124].

Several studies based on large-scale genome sequencing have been performed to identify the driver genes in carcinogenesis [125–128].

The objective was to detect the most frequently mutated genes among many different singular cases. However, identifying the driver genes in the long list of less frequent mutation proved difficult. One important new trend for delineating HCC biomarkers is the proteomic approach. It allows us to identify variations in levels of protein expression in liver tissue or plasma during the progression from liver fibrosis, cirrhosis or steatohepatitis to HCC [129]. The same approach was used with reference to molecular diagnosis and metastatic recurrence of HCC [130]. However, research focusing on the study of the pathogenesis of IM and MO by proteomic approach is at its beginning; studies are few and performed on a limited number of patients. Therefore, it is not currently possible to estimate whether the newly identified proteins are effectively potential biomarkers for identifying the multinodular HCCs of clonal origin and for discriminating between IM and MO cases.

Many efforts have also been dedicated to the exploration of new biologic mechanisms and molecular markers of multifocal HCC through omic analysis. The omic strategy includes the research of diagnostic and progression markers through genomic, proteomic and metabolomic analyses in order to evaluate gene, protein and metabolic deregulations. In this field, an undoubtedly innovative research has been recently published by Miao et al. [131], who performed a multi-omic analysis to differentiate MO from IM by decoding molecular differences between the two multifocal HCC models. This would allow us to identify molecular markers for diagnosis and prognosis, as well as therapeutic targets. They analyzed intrahepatic HCC lesions and matched non-cancerous liver tissue and blood obtained from representative patients with HBV-related multifocal HCC undergoing tumor resection and marked by distinct post-surgical courses. The samples were subjected to multi-omic analyses, integrating genomics and transcriptomics; the results, further validated by a cohort of 174 HCC patients, were correlated with clinicopathological data.

The determination of HBV integration in the different lesions clearly suggested the existence of different tumor clonality. The evaluation of genomic alterations showed how the enrichment of pathways including cell cycle, p53 signaling, histidine metabolism, G2/M checkpoint, and Ran (Ras-related nuclear protein)-mediated mitotic spindle regulation was associated with clonal metastasization rather than with the synchronous development of distinct clones. Protein analysis showed a significant difference in the synchronous development of multicentric primary HCC and metastatic disease. Validation analysis confirmed the upregulation of six out of seven genes: Histidine ammonia-lyase (HAL), stratifin 14-3-3γ (SFN), kinesin superfamily protein 15 (KIF15), dual-specificity protein kinase (TTK), Budding uninhibited by benzimidazoles 1 homolog (BUB1) and minichromosome maintenance complex component 4 (MCM4).

Different clinicopathologic features of HCCs were significantly associated with at least one of these genes. In addition, the evaluation of the relationships between the expression of the above genes and metastatic potential and postsurgical recurrence strongly suggested that TTK expression could be an independent prognostic indicator for HCC patients. In addition it could differentiate MO from IM. Multi-omic profiling could provide essential information for evaluating the aggressiveness of the existing lesion and for applying personalized therapies, including post-surgical treatments. It must be considered that cases of IM, with several nodules exhibiting different molecular alterations, require multi-omic analysis of each new nodule in order to identify critical molecular lesions which could be the targets of specific treatments.

Although the multi-omic strategy potentially opens new groundbreaking perspectives for diagnosis, prognosis and treatment of multifocal HCC, it still presents important limitations. The analysis should be extended to wider and more heterogeneous cohorts. Moreover, its clinical application could be seriously limited by the complexity of the analysis and by the elevated costs. Nonetheless, the innovative results of the multi-omic approach promotes new efforts to overcome these drawbacks.

REFERENCES

[1] El-Serag HB, Mason AC. Rising Incidence of Hepatocellular Carcinoma in the United States. *N Engl J Med.* 1999;340(10):745–50.

[2] Fan ST, Lo CM, Liu CL, Lam CM, Yuen WK, Yeung C, et al. Hepatectomy for hepatocellular carcinoma: toward zero hospital deaths. *Ann Surg.* 1999 Mar;229(3):322–30.

[3] Torzilli G. No-Mortality Liver Resection for Hepatocellular Carcinoma in Cirrhotic and Noncirrhotic Patients. *Arch Surg.* 1999;134(9):984.

[4] Belghiti J, Panis Y, Farges O, Benhamou JP, Fekete F. Intrahepatic recurrence after resection of hepatocellular carcinoma complicating cirrhosis. *Ann Surg.* 1991 Aug;214(2):114–7.

[5] Poon RT-P, Fan ST, Lo CM, Liu CL, Wong J. Long-term survival and pattern of recurrence after resection of small hepatocellular carcinoma in patients with preserved liver function: implications for a strategy of salvage transplantation. *Ann Surg.* 2002 Mar;235 (3):373–82.

[6] Marubashi S, Gotoh K, Akita H, Takahashi H, Sugimura K, Miyoshi N, et al. Analysis of Recurrence Patterns After Anatomical or Non-anatomical Resection for Hepatocellular Carcinoma. *Ann Surg Oncol.* 2015 Jul;22(7):2243–52.

[7] Ueno S, Kubo F, Sakoda M, Hiwatashi K, Tateno T, Mataki Y, et al. Efficacy of anatomic resection vs nonanatomic resection for small nodular hepatocellular carcinoma based on gross classification. *J Hepatobiliary Pancreat Surg.* 2008;15(5):493–500.

[8] Eguchi S, Kanematsu T, Arii S, Okazaki M, Okita K, Omata M, et al. Comparison of the outcomes between an anatomical subsegmentectomy and a non-anatomical minor hepatectomy for single hepatocellular carcinomas based on a Japanese nationwide survey. *Surgery.* 2008;143(4):469–75.

[9] Kobayashi A, Miyagawa S, Miwa S, Nakata T. Prognostic impact of anatomical resection on early and late intrahepatic recurrence in

patients with hepatocellular carcinoma. *J Hepatobiliary Pancreat Surg.* 2008 Oct 4;15(5):515–21.

[10] Wakai T, Shirai Y, Sakata J, Kaneko K, Cruz PV, Akazawa K, et al. Anatomic Resection Independently Improves Long-Term Survival in Patients with T1–T2 Hepatocellular Carcinoma. *Ann Surg Oncol.* 2007;14(4):1356–65.

[11] Makuuchi M, Imamura H, Sugawara Y, Takayama T. Progress in surgical treatment of hepatocellular carcinoma. *Oncology.* 2002;62 Suppl 1:74–81.

[12] Cucchetti A, Cescon M, Ercolani G, Bigonzi E, Torzilli G, Pinna AD. A comprehensive meta-regression analysis on outcome of anatomic resection versus nonanatomic resection for hepatocellular carcinoma. *Ann Surg Oncol.* 2012 Nov;19(12):3697–705.

[13] Kamiyama T, Nakanishi K, Yokoo H, Kamachi H, Matsushita M, Todo S. The impact of anatomical resection for hepatocellular carcinoma that meets the Milan criteria. *J Surg Oncol.* 2010 Jan 1;101(1):54–60.

[14] Yamazaki O, Matsuyama M, Horii K, Kanazawa A, Shimizu S, Uenishi T, et al. Comparison of the outcomes between anatomical resection and limited resection for single hepatocellular carcinomas no larger than 5 cm in diameter: a single-center study. *J Hepatobiliary Pancreat Sci.* 2010 May;17(3):349–58.

[15] Kaibori M, Kon M, Kitawaki T, Kawaura T, Hasegawa K, Kokudo N, et al. Comparison of anatomic and non-anatomic hepatic resection for hepatocellular carcinoma. *J Hepatobiliary Pancreat Sci.* 2017 Nov;24(11):616–26.

[16] Zhou Y, Xu D, Wu L, Li B. Meta-analysis of anatomic resection versus nonanatomic resection for hepatocellular carcinoma. *Langenbecks Arch Surg.* 2011 Oct;396(7):1109–17.

[17] Sakon M, Nagano H, Shimizu J, Kondo M, Nakamori S, Dono K, et al. Hepatic resection of hepatocellular carcinomas based on tumor hemodynamics. *J Surg Oncol.* 2000 Mar;73(3):179–81.

[18] Sakon M, Ogawa H, Fujita M, Nagano H. Hepatic resection for hepatocellular carcinoma based on tumor hemodynamics. *Hepatol Res.* 2012;43(2):155–64.

[19] Sakon M, Nagano H, Nakamori S, Dono K, Umeshita K, Murakami T, et al. Intrahepatic recurrences of hepatocellular carcinoma after hepatectomy: analysis based on tumor hemodynamics. *Arch Surg.* 2002 Jan;137(1):94–9.

[20] Xu W, Cao L, Chen L, Li J, Zhang XF, Qian HH, et al. Isolation of circulating tumor cells in patients with hepatocellular carcinoma using a novel cell separation strategy. *Clin Cancer Res.* 2011 Jun 1;17(11):3783–93.

[21] Funaki NO, Tanaka J, Seto SI, Kasamatsu T, Kaido T, Imamura M. Hematogenous spreading of hepatocellular carcinoma cells: possible participation in recurrence in the liver. *Hepatology.* 1997 Mar;25(3):564–8.

[22] Cho SH, Chun JM, Kwon HJ, Han YS, Kim SG, Hwang YJ. Outcomes and recurrence pattern after non-anatomic liver resection for solitary hepatocellular carcinomas. *Korean J Hepatobiliary Pancreat Surg.* 2016 Feb;20(1):1–7.

[23] Tanaka K, Shimada H, Matsumoto C, Matsuo K, Nagano Y, Endo I, et al. Anatomic versus limited nonanatomic resection for solitary hepatocellular carcinoma. *Surgery.* 2008;143(5):607–15.

[24] Kaibori M, Matsui Y, Hijikawa T, Uchida Y, Kwon AH, Kamiyama Y. Comparison of limited and anatomic hepatic resection for hepatocellular carcinoma with hepatitis C. *Surgery.* 2006 Mar;139(3):385–94.

[25] Okamura Y, Ito T, Sugiura T, Mori K, Uesaka K. Anatomic versus nonanatomichepatectomy for a solitary hepatocellular carcinoma: a case-controlled study with propensity score matching. *J Gastrointest Surg.* 2014 Nov;18(11):1994–2002.

[26] Nakashima T, Kojiro M. Pathologic Characteristics of Hepatocellular Carcinoma. *Semin Liver Dis.* 1986;6(03):259–66.

[27] Dutkowski P, Linecker M, DeOliveira ML, Müllhaupt B, Clavien PA. Challenges to liver transplantation and strategies to improve outcomes. *Gastroenterology.* 2015 Feb;148(2):307–23.

[28] Bruix J, Llovet JM. Prognostic prediction and treatment strategy in hepatocellular carcinoma. *Hepatology.* 2002 Mar;35(3):519–24.

[29] Llovet JM, Fuster J, Bruix J, of the Barcelona-Clinic Liver Cancer Group. The Barcelona approach: Diagnosis, staging, and treatment of hepatocellular carcinoma. *Liver Transpl.* 2004;10(S2):S115–20.

[30] Llovet J, Brú C, Bruix J. Prognosis of Hepatocellular Carcinoma: The BCLC Staging Classification. *Semin Liver Dis.* 1999;19 (03):329–38.

[31] Bruix J, Sherman M, Llovet JM, Beaugrand M, Lencioni R, Burroughs AK, et al. Clinical Management of Hepatocellular Carcinoma. Conclusions of the Barcelona-2000 EASL Conference. *J Hepatol.* 2001;35(3):421–30.

[32] Bruix J, Sherman M, American Association for the Study of Liver Diseases. Management of hepatocellular carcinoma: an update. *Hepatology.* 2011 Mar;53(3):1020–2.

[33] Cillo U, Vitale A, Grigoletto F, Farinati F, Brolese A, Zanus G, et al. Prospective validation of the Barcelona Clinic Liver Cancer staging system. *J Hepatol.* 2006 Apr;44(4):723–31.

[34] Marrero JA, Fontana RJ, Barrat A, Askari F, Conjeevaram HS, Su GL, et al. Prognosis of hepatocellular carcinoma: Comparison of 7 staging systems in an American cohort. *Hepatology.* 2005;41 (4):707–15.

[35] Ng KK, Vauthey JN, Pawlik TM, Lauwers GY, Regimbeau JM, Belghiti J, et al. Is Hepatic Resection for Large or Multinodular Hepatocellular Carcinoma Justified? Results from a Multi-Institutional Database. *Ann Surg Oncol.* 2005;12(5):364–73.

[36] Ishizawa T, Hasegawa K, Aoki T, Takahashi M, Inoue Y, Sano K, et al. Neither multiple tumors nor portal hypertension are surgical contraindications for hepatocellular carcinoma. *Gastroenterology.* 2008 Jun;134(7):1908–16.

[37] Torzilli G, Belghiti J, Kokudo N, Takayama T, Capussotti L, Nuzzo G, et al. A snapshot of the effective indications and results of surgery for hepatocellular carcinoma in tertiary referral centers: is it adherent to the EASL/AASLD recommendations?: an observational study of the HCC East-West study group. *Ann Surg.* 2013 May;257(5):929–37.

[38] Ciria R, López-Cillero P, Gallardo AB, Cabrera J, Pleguezuelo M, Ayllón MD, et al. Optimizing the management of patients with BCLC stage-B hepatocellular carcinoma: Modern surgical resection as a feasible alternative to transarterialchemoemolization. *Eur J Surg Oncol.* 2015 Sep;41(9):1153–61.

[39] Liang L, Xing H, Zhang H, Zhong J, Li C, Lau WY, et al. Surgical resection versus transarterial chemoembolization for BCLC intermediate stage hepatocellular carcinoma: a systematic review and meta-analysis. *HPB.* 2018 Feb;20(2):110–9.

[40] Bolondi L, Burroughs A, Dufour JF, Galle PR, Mazzaferro V, Piscaglia F, et al. Heterogeneity of patients with intermediate (BCLC B) Hepatocellular Carcinoma: proposal for a sub-classification to facilitate treatment decisions. *Semin Liver Dis.* 2012 Nov;32(4):348–59.

[41] Mazzaferro V, Llovet JM, Miceli R, Bhoori S, Schiavo M, Mariani L, et al. Predicting survival after liver transplantation in patients with hepatocellular carcinoma beyond the Milan criteria: a retrospective, exploratory analysis. *Lancet Oncol.* 2009 Jan;10(1):35–43.

[42] Li SQ, Huang T, Shen SL, Hua YP, Hu WJ, Kuang M, et al. Anatomical versus non-anatomicalliverresection for hepatocellular carcinoma exceeding Milan criteria. *Br J Surg.* 2017 Jan;104(1):118–27.

[43] Zoli M, Marchesini G, Melli A, Viti G, Marra A, Marrano D, et al. Evaluation of liver volume and liver function following hepatic resection in man. *Liver.* 1986 Oct;6(5):286–91.

[44] Asahara T, Dohi K, Katayama K, Itamoto T, Okamoto Y, Nakahara H, et al. Factors affecting postoperative prognosis in the solitary-

nodule type of hepatocellular carcinoma: experience of 132 cases in our institute. *Hiroshima J Med Sci.* 1998 Sep;47(3):99–104.

[45] Hirokawa F, Kubo S, Nagano H, Nakai T, Kaibori M, Hayashi M, et al. Do patients with small solitary hepatocellular carcinomas without macroscopically vascular invasion require anatomic resection? Propensity score analysis. *Surgery.* 2015 Jan;157(1):27–36.

[46] Park JH, Koh KC, Choi MS, Lee JH, Yoo BC, Paik SW, et al. Analysis of risk factors associated with early multinodular recurrences after hepatic resection for hepatocellular carcinoma. *Am J Surg*. 2006;192(1):29–33.

[47] Vauthey JN. Simplified Staging for Hepatocellular Carcinoma. *J Clin Oncol.* 2002;20(6):1527–36.

[48] Makuuchi M, Hasegawa H, Yamazaki S. Ultrasonically guided subsegmentectomy. *Surg Gynecol Obstet.* 1985;161:346–50.

[49] Helling TS, Blondeau B. Anatomic segmental resection compared to major hepatectomy in the treatment of liver neoplasms. *HPB.* 2005;7(3):222–5.

[50] Healey JE. Anatomy of the Biliary Ducts within the Human Liver. *AMA Arch Surg.* 1953;66(5):599.

[51] Couinaud C. *Le foie: études anatomiques et chirurgicales*. 1957. 530 p. [*The liver: anatomical and surgical studies*]

[52] Strasberg SM, Belghiti J, Clavien PA, Gadzijev E, Garden JO, Lau WY, et al. The Brisbane 2000 Terminology of Liver Anatomy and Resections. *HPB.* 2000;2(3):333–9.

[53] Ahn KS, Kang KJ, Park TJ, Kim YH, Lim TJ, Kwon JH. Benefit of Systematic Segmentectomy of the Hepatocellular Carcinoma. *Ann Surg*. 2013;258(6):1014–21.

[54] Takasaki K. Glissonean pedicle transection method for hepatic resection: a new concept of liver segmentation. *J Hepatobiliary Pancreat Surg*. 1998;5(3):286–91.

[55] Yamamoto M, Katagiri S, Ariizumi SI, Kotera Y, Takahashi Y. Glissonean pedicle transection method for liver surgery (with video). *J Hepatobiliary Pancreat Sci.* 2012 Jan;19(1):3–8.

[56] Ueno M, Hayami S, Sonomura T, Tanaka R, Kawai M, Hirono S, et al. Indocyanine green fluorescence imaging techniques and interventional radiology during laparoscopic anatomical liver resection (with video). *Surg Endosc.* 2017;32(2):1051–5.

[57] Takasaki K, Yamamoto M. Surgical Anatomy of the Liver in the Glissonean Pedicle Approach: What We Need to Know. In: *Venous Embolization of the Liver.* 2011. p. 23–7.

[58] Foster JH. Survival after liver resection for secondary tumors. *Am J Surg.* 1978;135(3):389–94.

[59] Lin TY, Chen KM, Liu TK. Total right hepatic lobectomy for primary hepatoma. *Surgery.* 1960 Dec;48:1048–60.

[60] Ton That Tung, Tung TT, Quang ND. A New Technique for Operating on the Liver. *Lancet.* 1963;281(7274):192–3.

[61] Bismuth H. Surgical anatomy and anatomical surgery of the liver. *World J Surg.* 1982 Jan;6(1):3–9.

[62] Couinaud CM. A simplified method for controlled left hepatectomy. *Surgery.* 1985 Mar;97(3):358–61.

[63] Couinaud C. Liver Anatomy: Portal (and Suprahepatic) or Biliary Segmentation. *Dig Surg.* 1999;16(6):459–67.

[64] Sugioka A, Kato Y, Tanahashi Y. Systematic extrahepatic Glissonean pedicle isolation for anatomical liver resection based on Laennec's capsule: proposal of a novel comprehensive surgical anatomy of the liver. *J Hepatobiliary Pancreat Sci.* 2017;24(1):17–23.

[65] Lee JH, Han DH, Jang DS, Choi GH, Choi JS. Robotic extrahepatic Glissonean pedicle approach for anatomic liver resection in the right liver: techniques and perioperative outcomes. *Surg Endosc.* 2016 Sep;30(9):3882–8.

[66] Ishizawa T, Saiura A, Kokudo N. Clinical application of indocyanine green-fluorescence imaging during hepatectomy. *Hepatobiliary Surg Nutr.* 2016 Aug;5(4):322–8.

[67] Aoki T, Yasuda D, Shimizu Y, Odaira M, Niiya T, Kusano T, et al. Image-guided liver mapping using fluorescence navigation system

with indocyanine green for anatomical hepatic resection. *World J Surg*. 2008 Aug;32(8):1763–7.

[68] Inoue Y, Arita J, Sakamoto T, Ono Y, Takahashi M, Takahashi Y, et al. Anatomical Liver Resections Guided by 3-Dimensional Parenchymal Staining Using Fusion Indocyanine Green Fluorescence Imaging. *Ann Surg*. 2015 Jul;262(1):105–11.

[69] Miyata A, Ishizawa T, Tani K, Shimizu A, Kaneko J, Aoki T, et al. Reappraisal of a Dye-Staining Technique for Anatomic Hepatectomy by the Concomitant Use of Indocyanine Green Fluorescence Imaging. *J Am Coll Surg*. 2015 Aug;221(2):e27–36.

[70] Ishizawa T, Zuker NB, Kokudo N, Gayet B. Positive and Negative Staining of Hepatic Segments by Use of Fluorescent Imaging Techniques During Laparoscopic Hepatectomy. *Arch Surg* [Internet]. 2012;147(4). Available from: http://dx.doi.org/10.1001/archsurg.2012.59.

[71] Inoue Y, Saiura A, Arita J, Takahashi Y. Hepatic Vein-Oriented Liver Resection Using Fusion Indocyanine Green Fluorescence Imaging. *Ann Surg*. 2015 Dec;262(6):e98–9.

[72] Ishizawa T, Gumbs AA, Kokudo N, Gayet B. Laparoscopic segmentectomy of the liver: from segment I to VIII. *Ann Surg*. 2012 Dec;256(6):959–64.

[73] Viganò L, Russolillo N, Ferrero A, Langella S, Sperti E, Capussotti L. Evolution of long-term outcome of liver resection for colorectal metastases: analysis of actual 5-year survival rates over two decades. *Ann Surg Oncol*. 2012 Jun;19(6):2035–44.

[74] Sahani DV, Bajwa MA, Andrabi Y, Bajpai S, Cusack JC. Current status of imaging and emerging techniques to evaluate liver metastases from colorectal carcinoma. *Ann Surg*. 2014 May;259(5):861–72.

[75] Lang H, Radtke A, Liu C, Frühauf N, Peitgen H, Broelsch C. Extended left hepatectomy?modified operation planning based on three-dimensional visualization of liver anatomy. *Langenbecks Arch Surg* [Internet]. 2003;389(4). Available from: http://dx.doi.org/10.1007/s00423-003-0441-z.

[76] Kishi Y, Abdalla EK, Chun YS, Zorzi D, Madoff DC, Wallace MJ, et al. Three hundred and one consecutive extended right hepatectomies: evaluation of outcome based on systematic liver volumetry. *Ann Surg*. 2009 Oct;250(4):540–8.

[77] Donadon M, Costa G, Torzilli G. State of the art of intraoperative ultrasound in liver surgery: current use for staging and resection guidance. *Ultraschall Med.* 2014 Dec;35(6):500–11; quiz 512–3.

[78] Lai EC, Fan ST, Lo CM, Chu KM, Liu CL, Wong J. Hepatic resection for hepatocellular carcinoma. An audit of 343 patients. *Ann Surg*. 1995 Mar;221(3):291–8.

[79] Colecchia A, Schiumerini R, Cucchetti A, Cescon M, Taddia M, Marasco G, et al. Prognostic factors for hepatocellular carcinoma recurrence. *World J Gastroenterol.* 2014 May 28;20(20):5935–50.

[80] Shim JH, Jun MJ, Han S, Lee YJ, Lee SG, Kim KM, et al. Prognostic nomograms for prediction of recurrence and survival after curative liver resection for hepatocellular carcinoma. *Ann Surg*. 2015 May;261(5):939–46.

[81] Kamiyama T, Nakanishi K, Yokoo H, Kamachi H, Tahara M, Kakisaka T, et al. Analysis of the risk factors for early death due to disease recurrence or progression within 1 year after hepatectomy in patients with hepatocellular carcinoma. *World J Surg Oncol.* 2012 Jun 14;10:107.

[82] Yamanaka N, Okamoto E, Kawamura E, Kato T, Oriyama T, Fujimoto J, et al. Dynamics of normal and injured human liver regeneration after hepatectomy as assessed on the basis of computed tomography and liver function. *Hepatology.* 1993 Jul;18(1):79–85.

[83] Yasui M, Harada A, Torii A, Nakao A, Nonami T, Takagi H. Impaired liver function and long-term prognosis after hepatectomy for hepatocellular carcinoma. *World J Surg*. 1995;19(3):439–43.

[84] Eguchi S, Kanematsu T, Arii S, Okazaki M, Okita K, Omata M, et al. Comparison of the outcomes between an anatomical subsegmentectomy and a non-anatomical minor hepatectomy for

single hepatocellular carcinomas based on a Japanese nationwide survey. *Surgery.* 2008;143(4):469–75.

[85] Hasegawa K, Kokudo N, Imamura H, Matsuyama Y, Aoki T, Minagawa M, et al. Prognostic impact of anatomic resection for hepatocellular carcinoma. *Ann Surg.* 2005 Aug;242(2):252–9.

[86] Cucchetti A, Qiao GL, Cescon M, Li J, Xia Y, Ercolani G, et al. Anatomic versus nonanatomic resection in cirrhotic patients with early hepatocellular carcinoma. *Surgery.* 2014 Mar;155(3):512–21.

[87] Yan L. *Operative Techniques in Liver Resection.* Springer; 2015. 354 p.

[88] Shindoh J, Makuuchi M, Matsuyama Y, Mise Y, Arita J, Sakamoto Y, et al. Complete removal of the tumor-bearing portal territory decreases local tumor recurrence and improves disease-specific survival of patients with hepatocellular carcinoma. *J Hepatol.* 2016 Mar;64(3):594–600.

[89] Marubashi S, Gotoh K, Akita H, Takahashi H, Ito Y, Yano M, et al. Anatomical versus non-anatomical resection for hepatocellular carcinoma. *Br J Surg.* 2015 Jun;102(7):776–84.

[90] Yamamoto T, Yagi S, Uryuhara K, Kaihara S, Hosotani R. Clinical factors that affect the outcomes after anatomical versus non-anatomical resection for hepatocellular carcinoma. *Surg Today.* 2017 Feb;47(2):193–201.

[91] Miyagawa S, Kawasaki S, Makuuchi M. Comparison of the characteristics of hepatocellular carcinoma between hepatitis B and C viral infection: tumor multicentricity in cirrhotic liver with hepatitis C. *Hepatology.* 1996 Aug;24(2):307–10.

[92] Kim BK, Han KH, Park YN, Park MS, Kim KS, Choi JS, et al. Prediction of microvascular invasion before curative resection of hepatocellular carcinoma. *J Surg Oncol.* 2008 Mar 1;97(3):246–52.

[93] Pawlik TM, Delman KA, Vauthey JN, Nagorney DM, Ng IOL, Ikai I, et al. Tumor size predicts vascular invasion and histologic grade: Implications for selection of surgical treatment for hepatocellular carcinoma. *Liver Transpl.* 2005 Sep;11(9):1086–92.

[94] Marubashi S, Gotoh K, Akita H, Takahashi H, Sugimura K, Miyoshi N, et al. Analysis of Recurrence Patterns After Anatomical or Non-anatomical Resection for Hepatocellular Carcinoma. *Ann Surg Oncol.* 2014;22(7):2243–52.

[95] Tomimaru Y, Eguchi H, Marubashi S, Wada H, Kobayashi S, Tanemura M, et al. Equivalent outcomes after anatomical and non-anatomical resection of small hepatocellular carcinoma in patients with preserved liver function. *Dig Dis Sci.* 2012 Jul;57(7):1942–8.

[96] Sasaki K, Shindoh J, Margonis GA, Nishioka Y, Andreatos N, Sekine A, et al. Effect of Background Liver Cirrhosis on Outcomes of Hepatectomy for Hepatocellular Carcinoma. *JAMA Surg.* 2017 Mar 15;152(3):e165059.

[97] Sakamoto M, Hirohashi S, Tsuda H, Shimosato Y, Makuuchi M, Hosoda Y. Multicentric independent development of hepatocellular carcinoma revealed by analysis of hepatitis B virus integration pattern. *Am J Surg Pathol.* 1989 Dec;13(12):1064–7.

[98] Morimoto O, Nagano H, Sakon M, Fujiwara Y, Yamada T, Nakagawa H, et al. Diagnosis of intrahepatic metastasis and multicentric carcinogenesis by microsatellite loss of heterozygosity in patients with multiple and recurrent hepatocellular carcinomas. *J Hepatol.* 2003 Aug;39(2):215–21.

[99] Li Q, Wang J, Juzi JT, Sun Y, Zheng H, Cui Y, et al. Clonality analysis for multicentric origin and intrahepatic metastasis in recurrent and primary hepatocellular carcinoma. *J Gastrointest Surg.* 2008 Sep;12(9):1540–7.

[100] Yang SL, Luo YY, Chen M, Zhou YP, Lu FR, Deng DF, et al. A systematic review and meta-analysis comparing the prognosis of multicentric occurrence and vs. intrahepatic metastasis in patients with recurrent hepatocellular carcinoma after hepatectomy. *HPB.* 2017 Oct;19(10):835–42.

[101] Zhou L, Rui JA, Wang SB, Chen SG, Qu Q. Early recurrence in large hepatocellular carcinoma after curative hepatic resection: prognostic significance and risk factors. *Hepatogastroenterology.* 2014 Oct;61(135):2035–41.

[102] Hung HH, Lei HJ, Chau GY, Su CW, Hsia CY, Kao WY, et al. Milan criteria, multi-nodularity, and microvascular invasion predict the recurrence patterns of hepatocellular carcinoma after resection. *J Gastrointest Surg.* 2013 Apr;17(4):702–11.

[103] Hirokawa F, Hayashi M, Asakuma M, Shimizu T, Inoue Y, Uchiyama K. Risk factors and patterns of early recurrence after curative hepatectomy for hepatocellular carcinoma. *Surg Oncol.* 2016 Mar;25(1):24–9.

[104] Zhong Y, Deng M, Xu R. Reappraisal of evidence of microscopic portal vein involvement by hepatocellular carcinoma cells with stratification of tumor size. *World J Surg.* 2015 May;39(5):1142–9.

[105] Regimbeau JM, Kianmanesh R, Farges O, Dondero F, Sauvanet A, Belghiti J. Extent of liver resection influences the outcome in patients with cirrhosis and small hepatocellular carcinoma. *Surgery.* 2002;131(3):311–7.

[106] Hasegawa K, Kokudo N, Imamura H, Matsuyama Y, Aoki T, Minagawa M, et al. Prognostic Impact of Anatomic Resection for Hepatocellular Carcinoma. *Ann Surg.* 2005;242(2):252–9.

[107] Takano S, Oishi H, Kono S, Kawakami S, Nakamura M, Kubota N, et al. Retrospective analysis of type of hepatic resection for hepatocellular carcinoma. *Br J Surg.* 2000 Jan;87(1):65–70.

[108] Ercolani G, Grazi GL, Ravaioli M, Del Gaudio M, Gardini A, Cescon M, et al. Liver resection for hepatocellular carcinoma on cirrhosis: univariate and multivariate analysis of risk factors for intrahepatic recurrence. *Ann Surg.* 2003 Apr;237(4):536–43.

[109] Cucchetti A, Qiao GL, Cescon M, Li J, Xia Y, Ercolani G, et al. Anatomic versus nonanatomic resection in cirrhotic patients with early hepatocellular carcinoma. *Surgery.* 2014 Mar;155(3):512–21.

[110] Li SL, Su M, Peng T, Xiao KY, Shang LM, Xu BH, et al. Clinicopathologic Characteristics and Prognoses for Multicentric Occurrence and Intrahepatic Metastasis in Synchronous Multinodular Hepatocellular Carcinoma Patients. *Asian Pac J Cancer Prev.* 2013;14(1):217–23.

[111] Shimada M, Hamatsu T, Yamashita Y, Rikimaru T, Taguchi K, Utsunomiya T, et al. Characteristics of multicentric hepatocellular carcinomas: comparison with intrahepatic metastasis. *World J Surg.* 2001 Aug;25(8):991–5.

[112] Nakano S, Haratake J, Okamoto K, Takeda S. Investigation of resected multinodular hepatocellular carcinoma: assessment of unicentric or multicentric genesis from histological and prognostic viewpoint. *Am J Gastroenterol.* 1994 Feb;89(2):189–93.

[113] Ikeda K, Arase Y, Kobayashi M, Saitoh S, Someya T, Hosaka T, et al. Significance of multicentric cancer recurrence after potentially curative ablation of hepatocellular carcinoma: a long term cohort study of 892 patients with viral cirrhosis. *J Gastroenterol.* 2003;38(9):865–76.

[114] Arii S, Yamaoka Y, Futagawa S, Inoue K, Kobayashi K, Kojiro M, et al. Results of surgical and nonsurgical treatment for small-sized hepatocellular carcinomas: A retrospective and nationwide survey in Japan. *Hepatology.* 2000;32(6):1224–9.

[115] Huang ZY, Liang BY, Xiong M, Zhan DQ, Wei S, Wang GP, et al. Long-term outcomes of repeat hepatic resection in patients with recurrent hepatocellular carcinoma and analysis of recurrent types and their prognosis: a single-center experience in China. *Ann Surg Oncol*. 2012 Aug;19(8):2515–25.

[116] Portolani N, Coniglio A, Ghidoni S, Giovanelli M, Benetti A, Tiberio GAM, et al. Early and late recurrence after liver resection for hepatocellular carcinoma: prognostic and therapeutic implications. *Ann Surg.* 2006 Feb;243(2):229–35.

[117] Frau M, Feo F, Pascale RM. Pleiotropic effects of methionine adenosyltransferases deregulation as determinants of liver cancer progression and prognosis. *J Hepatol.* 2013 Oct;59(4):830–41.

[118] Calvisi DF, Frau M, Tomasi ML, Feo F, Pascale RM. Deregulation of signalling pathways in prognostic subtypes of hepatocellular carcinoma: novel insights from interspecies comparison. *Biochim Biophys Acta.* 2012 Aug;1826(1):215–37.

[119] Lam CT, Tang CMC, Lau KW, Lung ML. Loss of heterozygosity on chromosome 11 in esophageal squamous cell carcinomas. *Cancer Lett.* 2002;178(1):75–81.

[120] Piao Z, Kim H, Malkhosyan S, Park C. Frequent chromosomal instability but no microsatellite instability in hepatocellular carcinomas. *Int J Oncol* [Internet]. 2000; Available from: http://dx.doi.org/10.3892/ijo.17.3.507.

[121] Chen YJ, Yeh SH, Chen JT, Wu CC, Hsu MT, Tsai SF, et al. Chromosomal changes and clonality relationship between primary and recurrent hepatocellular carcinoma. *Gastroenterology.* 2000 Aug;119(2):431–40.

[122] Ng IOL, Guan XY, Poon RTP, Fan ST, Lee JMF. Determination of the molecular relationship between multiple tumour nodules in hepatocellular carcinoma differentiates multicentric origin from intrahepatic metastasis. *J Pathol.* 2003 Mar;199(3):345–53.

[123] Utsunomiya T, Shimada M, Imura S, Morine Y, Ikemoto T, Mori M. Molecular signatures of noncancerous liver tissue can predict the risk for late recurrence of hepatocellular carcinoma. *J Gastroenterol.* 2010 Feb;45(2):146–52.

[124] Nakata T, Seki N, Miwa S, Kobayashi A, Soeda J, Nimura Y, et al. Identification of genes associated with multiple nodules in hepatocellular carcinoma using cDNA microarray: multicentric occurrence or intrahepatic metastasis? *Hepatogastroenterology.* 2008 May;55(84):865–72.

[125] Fujimoto A, Totoki Y, Abe T, Boroevich KA, Hosoda F, Nguyen HH, et al. Whole-genome sequencing of liver cancers identifies etiological influences on mutation patterns and recurrent mutations in chromatin regulators. *Nat Genet.* 2012;44(7):760–4.

[126] Totoki Y, Tatsuno K, Yamamoto S, Arai Y, Hosoda F, Ishikawa S, et al. High-resolution characterization of a hepatocellular carcinoma genome. *Nat Genet.* 2011 May;43(5):464–9.

[127] Guichard C, Amaddeo G, Imbeaud S, Ladeiro Y, Pelletier L, Ben Maad I, et al. Integrated analysis of somatic mutations and focal

copy-number changes identifies key genes and pathways in hepatocellular carcinoma. *Nat Genet.* 2012;44(6):694–8.

[128] Furuta M, Ueno M, Fujimoto A, Hayami S, Yasukawa S, Kojima F, et al. Whole genome sequencing discriminates hepatocellular carcinoma with intrahepatic metastasis from multi-centric tumors. *J Hepatol.* 2017;66(2):363–73.

[129] Beretta L. Comparative analysis of the liver and plasma proteomes as a novel and powerful strategy for hepatocellular carcinoma biomarker discovery. *Cancer Lett.* 2009 Dec 1;286(1):134–9.

[130] Qin LX, Tang ZY. Recent progress in predictive biomarkers for metastatic recurrence of human hepatocellular carcinoma: a review of the literature. *J Cancer Res Clin Oncol.* 2004 Sep;130(9):497–513.

[131] Miao R, Luo H, Zhou H, Li G, Bu D, Yang X, et al. Identification of prognostic biomarkers in hepatitis B virus-related hepatocellular carcinoma and stratification by integrative multi-omics analysis. *J Hepatol.* 2014 Oct;61(4):840–9.

In: Handbook of Surgical Procedures
Editor: Heather Gilbert
ISBN: 978-1-53614-580-9

Chapter 2

LAPAROSCOPIC LIVER RESECTION FOR HEPATOCELLULAR CARCINOMA PATIENTS: INDICATIONS AND BENEFITS

Zenichi Morise*[*], *MD, PhD, FACS
Professor, Department of Surgery,
Fujita Health University School of Medicine
Toyoake, Japan

ABSTRACT

The treatment options for hepatocellular carcinoma (HCC) include liver resection (LR), liver transplantation (LT), transarterial chemo-embolization, and local ablation therapy. LR and LT, and local ablation therapy (for small tumors only) provide the best hope for cure. However, most patients with HCC have underlying chronic liver disease (CLD) and are thus at high risk for development of postoperative complications - sometimes fatal- and metachronous multicentric recurrent lesions occurring from the preneoplastic CLD background. Although appropriate treatment is selected for HCC patients with CLD depending on the tumor

[*] Corresponding Author Email: zmorise@fujita-hu.ac.jp.

condition and liver function, a large number of patients are not able to undergo any treatment because of poor liver function and/or complicated tumor condition. This is especially true after repeated treatments for the disease.

In our experience of laparoscopic LR (LLR), LLR could expand the indication of LR to severe CLD patients due to its lower damages to the liver and surrounding tissue, especially to collateral circulation around the cirrhotic liver. Child-Pugh score, not class, is one of the promising candidates as a selection indicator which correlates well to our indication criteria of surface small LLR to severe CLD patients, patient's performance status, and prognosis. Portal hypertension should also be counted in the selection criteria.

For repeat LLR, there are only small number of reports with small number of patients to date. These studies generally reported that repeat LLR has better short-term outcomes than open (reduced bleedings, less or similar morbidity and shorter hospital stay) without compromising the long-term outcomes. The fact that complete adhesiolysis can be avoided in repeat LLR is also reported. In the comparison of previous procedures, it is reported that the operation time for repeat LLR was shorter for the patients previously treated with LLR than open. Furthermore, it is speculated that LLR for minor repeat LR of cirrhotic liver can be minimized the deterioration of liver function by LR. However, further experience and evaluation of anatomical resection or resections exposing major vessels as repeat LLR, especially after previous anatomical resection, are needed.

It is thought that the features of LLR could lead to expanding the indications for LR to those patients in the settings of severe CLD, repeat LR, and bridging to LT. There should be a chance to prolong the overall survival of the patients by using LLR as a powerful local therapy which can be applied repeatedly with minimal deterioration of liver function.

INTRODUCTION

General Situation of the Treatments for Hepatocellular Carcinoma (HCC) Patients with Chronic Liver Disease (CLD)

The treatment options for HCC include liver resection (LR) [1], liver transplantation (LT) [2], transarterial chemoembolization, and local ablation therapy [3]. LR, LT and local ablation therapy (only for small tumors) provide the best hope for cure [3-6]. However, most patients with

HCC have underlying chronic liver disease (CLD) and are thus at high risk for development of postoperative complications and metachronous multicentric recurrent lesions occurring from the preneoplastic CLD background.

Currently, the choice of LR, LT, local ablation therapy or transarterial chemoembolization is made for each patient depending on the tumor condition and liver function [7]. However, a large number of HCC patients are not able to undergo any such treatment because of poor liver function and/or complicated tumor condition. This is especially true after repeated treatments for the recurrent disease.

Among the treatment options mentioned above, LT should be ideal for HCC patients with CLD in the aspect of removing both existing tumors and injured/preneoplastic underlying liver. However, it cannot be applied on a large scale due to the high prevalence of HCC and the limited access to LT consequent to donor shortage [8]. LT is also restricted to patients with minimal risk of tumor recurrence under immunosuppression [9]. Expansion of the criteria for LT in HCC patients is still under trial and discussion [10, 11]. Therefore, LR has traditionally been accepted as the preferred treatment for resectable HCC in patients with adequate liver reserve [6, 12, 13].

When considering LR to HCC patients with CLD, not only the oncological therapeutic effects, but also the residual liver function and the degree of invasive surgical stress, especially to the diseased liver should be considered. Patients with CLD have various symptoms [14] and a high risk of morbidity and mortality following anesthesia and surgery depending on their Child-Pugh (CP) class [15, 16]. For severe CLD patients, even limited LR often leads to refractory ascites, which can be a fatal complication [17, 18].

Considerable progress made over the past 10 years in screening, early radiologic diagnosis, treatment of the underlying CLD, and surgical techniques has resulted in revision of the indications for LR [19]. Furthermore, improved liver function assessment and understanding of segmental liver anatomy from using more accurate imaging studies, as well as surgical technical progress, are the most important factors that have reduced the mortality rate of HCC; today, the expected 5-year survival after LR is 38%-61%, depending on the stage of the disease [20]. Despite these advances, however, less than 30% of HCC patients are eligible for LR [21, 22].

Emerging evidence from laparoscopic (L)LR [23, 24] may lead to expansion of the indication for LR in the therapeutic system for HCC patients with CLD. In this article, the current reports on LLR for HCC patients with CLD are reviewed and our experiences are described.

LLR for HCC Patients with CLD

The beginnings of LLR were at the start of the 1990s, with its initial reports [25-27] being published in 1991 and 1992. Thereafter, the indication of LLR has been expanded as a less invasive procedure than conventional open (O)LR for hepatic lesions. LLR has the benefit of earlier intake, recovery and discharge, and reduced postoperative pain, like other laparoscopic procedures [28]. A meta-analysis of 26 studies found that, although LLR was associated with longer operating times, the oncologic outcomes were not different from OLR [29]. Furthermore, studies showed the specific advantages associated with LLR, such as reduced blood loss, decreased portal clamp time, and decreases in overall and liver-specific complications at least for selected patients and within the technical capabilities of each experienced center.

The safety and feasibility of LLR and its short-term benefits for HCC patients with CLD have also been demonstrated [30-32]. LLR may be particularly advantageous for HCC patients with CLD, who often develop refractory ascites with OLR, a potentially fatal complication [17, 18]. LLR has the advantage of minimal ascites, due to the preservation of venous and lymphatic collateral circulation [35], which lowers the risk of water/electrolyte imbalance and hypoproteinemia that could trigger fatal liver failure. This feature could be the most remarkable advantage of LLR.

Patients who undergo LR are exposed to three different types of stresses: 1) general, whole-body surgical stress; 2) reduced liver function due to reduced liver volume after resection; and, (3) surgery-induced injury to the environment surrounding the liver and liver parenchyma (caused by disruption of the collateral blood and lymphatic circulation with laparotomy and mobilization of the liver, and parenchymal injury by compression of the liver) [33]. LR is the procedure that the liver protected inside the subphrenic rib cage is resected. In OLR, the cage is opened with a big subcostal incision and a lift of the costal arch, and then the liver is picked up for resection with the dissection of retroperitoneal attachments. On the other, in LLR, laparoscope and forceps intrude into the cage directly from the caudal direction ("Caudal approach" [34-36], Figure 1) and perform LR in the small targeted area without damages to the surrounding area. Furthermore, the same surgical view under position changes, acquired by the adjustments of laparoscope's positioning and rotation in LLR, allows for handling large-volume liver/tumor by postural changes. This leads to the reduction of compression damage on the liver. Our previous report of the caudal approach posterior sectionectomy in the left lateral position [34] posed the novel concept of "caudal approach" in LLR. Although the supine to semi-lateral positioning had been employed for the other resections, the transection plane of posterior sectionectomy was horizontal in the supine position and gravity obstructs the exposure of the plane. A clear view from the caudal direction and an easy access to postural changes are among the advantages of LLR (Figure 1). Our procedure is a laparoscopic posterior sectionectomy with parenchymal transection prior to mobilization in the left lateral position. It facilitates exposure of the cutting plane during the transection in caudal-to-cranial one direction. The transection plane is well-opened between the retroperitoneal-fixed posterior section and the remnant liver falling down to left by gravity. Moreover, the segmentectomy or partial resection of segment (S)7 should be performed in the deeper and smaller cranial subphrenic space and S6 is an obstacle under the laparoscopic caudal view even in the left lateral position. We employed the semi-prone position with only partial dissection of the retroperitoneum for those resections [37]. LLR can facilitate minimal dissection around the liver and minimal compression on the liver with the intrusion and manipulation of laparoscope and forceps to the small target area ("Caudal approach" Figure 1) under postural changes. Therefore, LLR's reduction of surgery-induced injuries in HCC patients with CLD lowers the risk of refractory ascites, resulting in a reduced risk of successive complications and facilitating a smoother recovery without liver failure.

The impact of LLR on this issue should depend on the severity of the background CLD, the operative technique (extent of dissection of the peritoneal attachments and adhesions), and extent of resection. Our previous study compared the short-term results of liver surface small LLR for patients with severe CLD (CP-B/C and indocyanine green retention rate at 15 min (ICGR15) $\geq$ 40%) to those for patients with mild-moderate CLD [38]. Although the study was a small number, retrospective unmatched study, it revealed comparable perioperative outcomes, including postoperative ascites production, between patients with severe and mild-to-moderate CLD in LLR.

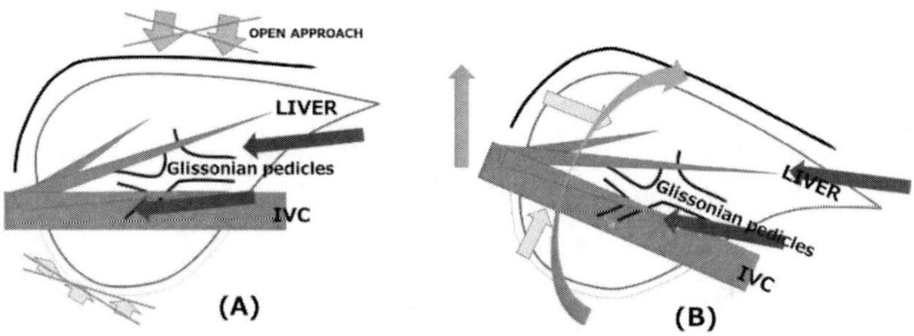

Figure 1 Schema of laparoscopic liver resection (LLR, A), and position changes in LLR (B). Red arrows indicate the directions of the view and manipulation. In the open approach, the subcostal cage containing the liver is opened with a large subcostal incision, and instruments are used to lift the costal arch up (A, cross mark). The liver is dissected and mobilized (picked up) from the retroperitoneum (A, cross mark).
A: In the laparoscopic caudal approach, the laparoscope and forceps intrude into the subcostal cage from caudal direction, and surgery is performed with minimal alteration and destruction of the surrounding structures. B: In the laparoscopic approach, the same surgical view under position changes (tilting the bed and rotation of the patient's body), acquired by the adjustments of laparoscope's positioning and rotation, allows for handling large-volume liver/tumor by postural changes.

Repeat LLR

As mentioned above, HCC arises in metachronous multicentric fashion inside the liver with its preneoplastic CLD backgrounds. Intrahepatic recurrences after previous resection of HCC with the need for repeat treatments often occur.

LR is now actively applied to those lesions, when the lesions are resectable and there is no other uncontrollable/distant disease, and the opportunity for repeat LR has increased [39-42]. Currently, indications of LLR have been expanded with the accumulation of experiences and technical/conceptual and instrumental developments [24, 43-45]. Postoperative adhesions with the need for adhesiolysis are known to increase the operation time of subsequent surgeries and the incidence of bowel injury [46, 47]. Therefore, increased rates of complications and conversion from laparoscopic to open surgery had been reported in repeat laparoscopic surgery [48]. Although a previous surgical history had been among the contraindications for laparoscopic surgery, many laparoscopic procedures, such as cholecystectomy [47, 48], appendectomy [49], colectomy [50], and gastrectomy [51], can be applied to those patients nowadays with technical and instrumental improvements. However, since LLR still remains a technically demanding procedure, the indications and efficacy of repeat LLR are under discussion. Adequate dissection of adhesion and mobilization of the involved liver should be performed before repeat LR. Visualization and dissection of the hepatoduodenal ligament and hilar area, often crucial in LR, can be disrupted by adhesion. The deformity of the liver surrounded by the scars and adhesion makes the localization of tumors and the important structures (vessels) difficult. The fact that liver capsule bleeds easily during adhesiolysis and mobilization leads to increase the intraoperative bleeding and create a suboptimal operative field [52]. These changes after previous surgery can increase the risks of intraoperative injury to vascular and biliary structures.

Although the reports of repeat LLR are gradually increasing, only 16 reports of small series were found out under Medline-search with the words “repeat” and “laparoscopic liver resection” and their re-quotations

[53-68]. Belli et al. [55] reported that LLR facilitates more meticulous dissection of adhesions strained by the pneumoperitoneum using magnified laparoscopic view. The fact that complete adhesiolysis can be avoided when the adhesion does not affect the current operative procedure (which is on the same line of LLR characteristics mentioned in the previous section "LLR for HCC patients with CLD") is also reported as a possible advantage of repeat LLR [59, 64]. In comparison with repeat OLR, these studies generally reported that repeat LLR has better short-term outcomes (similar or longer operation time, reduced bleedings, reduced blood transfusion rate, less or similar morbidity and shorter hospital stay) without compromising the long-term outcomes. Each report concluded that repeat LLR is feasible and safe for selected patients. However, those studies are the mixtures of the patients with HCC and metastases. Five studies of repeat LLR, which only include HCC patients [55, 59, 61, 62, 66], reported the outcomes for the series of 12, 6, 3, 20 and 8 patients. The conclusions of all studies are that repeat LLR is a safe and feasible procedure even for recurrent HCC in CLD patients. Belli et al. [55] again mentioned that the adhesiolysis was easier and the operation time was shorter in repeat LLR for the patients with previous LLR compared to previous OLR. They also referred the advantages of LLR for the management during the long history with repeat oncogenesis in CLD patients. Kanazawa et al. [62] mentioned that the complication rate and the hospital stay had been decreased in their institute by the introduction of LLR for recurrent HCC patients. Repeat LLR requires smaller (than open) working space between adhesions where laparoscope and forceps can intrude and do manipulation. This fact allows for minimal adhesiolysis and a direct approach to the tumor especially in repeat small LLR [58, 59, 64]. Therefore, some studies showed that operation time and bleeding amount were similar in primary and repeat LLR [53, 64], although the short-term results from primary and repeat OLR are usually very different especially in operative time (longer in repeat) and intraoperative blood loss (larger in repeat). Operation time and bleeding amount could be reduced with the usage of laparoscopic approach for repeat partial resection. Furthermore, one of the possible advantages

speculated for minor repeat LLR of CLD liver is that the deterioration of liver function can be minimized with the minimal dissection (Table 1).

LLR Indications to Severe CLD Patients

For the treatment selection of HCC, the Barcelona clinic liver cancer (BCLC) staging system/treatment algorithm [69] and the Japan Society of Hepatology clinical guidelines for HCC (JSH guideline) [70] are used in Western countries and Japan, respectively. Both systems include not only tumor condition but also background liver condition for the treatment selection. The two differ in that the BCLC algorithm uses CP classification (CP) [71] for assessments of liver function, while the JSH guideline uses the liver damage (LD) classification of the Liver Cancer Study Group of Japan [72], which has ICGR15 as one of the essential elements.

Table 1. The summary of present status of repeat LLR

- Operation time was shorter and the adhesiolysis was easier for the patients previously treated with LLR than open LR.
- LLR facilitates more meticulous dissection of adhesions strained by the pneumoperitoneum using magnified laparoscopic view.
- Complete adhesiolysis can be avoided in repeat LLR when the adhesion does not affect the current operative procedure, since it requires smaller (than open) working space between adhesions. (This allows that operation time and bleeding amount are similar to primary LLR, although those from open LR are longer and larger.)

LLR could prolong the overall survival of the HCC patients with CLD as a powerful local therapy which can be applied repeatedly with minimal deterioration of liver function.

Challenges:

Further evaluations of anatomical resection or resections exposing major vessels after previous anatomical resection are needed.

ICGR15 is a useful modality for assessing hepatic functional reserve and predicting postoperative mortality [73-75]. The extent of the liver resected in each patient is basically planned according to the tumor condition and location. However, HCC patients sometimes develop postoperative liver failure due to poor liver functional reserve after the planned resection. ICGR15 has been an excellent tool for predicting how much liver volume could be resected in each patient's liver condition [74], On the other hand, nontumorous functioning liver parenchyma is resected minimally in liver surface tumorectomy or small partial resection. In those cases, the most important point for preoperative evaluation is, not how much liver volume could be resected, but whether the patient and the liver could tolerate the surgical stress. As mentioned before, LLR minimizes the surgery-induced injury caused by disruption of the collateral blood and lymphatic circulation and compression on the liver parenchyma, and leads to decreased postoperative ascites and liver failure [33]. The decision-making process during liver surface small partial LLR should be different from the other liver resections.

Our Experiences of LLR for HCC Patients with CLD

Among 152 patients, 19 had more than 30% ICGR15 and HCC. The details of these patients are presented in Table 2. The 19 patients were composed of 6, 11 and 2 patients with CP-A, B and C, respectively. By LD classification, they included 2, 12 and 5 patients of LD-A, B and C, respectively. There was discrepancy between the liver functional assessments of CP and LD. The patients with high ICGR15 values tended to be classified into higher grade of liver dysfunction in the LD classification. Based on liver functional criteria only of BCLC and JHS, there were already 2 and 5 patients out of LR indication in this group, respectively. We applied liver surface small LLR to the CP-B/C (up to CP score of 10) patients only when the patients could have been doing light or household labor for more than 6 months before their surgery, in a stable condition (good performance status).

Table 2. Our cases of laparoscopic liver resection (LLR) for severe chronic liver diseases (CLD)

Age	Sex	Tumor location	Tumor size (mm)	Conversion	Previous surgery	LT after LLR	ICGR15 (%)	CP		Platelet ($X10^4/\mu l$)	Prognosis (month)	
73	F	S3	18				37.7	A	6	14.7	5	A
66	M	S3	47		Splenectomy		31.1	B	7	26	5.1	D
53	M	S5-6	28				41.2	B	7	8.3	11.2	D
63	M	S5-6	40				52	B	9	4.5	12	D
68	F	S8	13				58.2	C	10	4	14.1	D
75	F	S3	20				42.5	B	9	5.8	17.4	D
67	M	S8	20	HALS			55	B	8	5	19.3	D
69	F	S8	24		LLR		33.5	B	7	5.8	22.7	D
72	M	S5	16		LLR		42.3	A	5	8.6	27.8	A
64	M	S4,S2-3	41				42.8	B	7	8.9	28.5	D
81	F	S7	100				78.3	A	5	36.6	28.6	A
62	M	S3	24		LLRX3		43.5	B	8	7.2	30.5	A
68	F	S4	23				40	B	9	6.7	35.4	D
80	F	S3	18		LLR		40.4	B	7	8.8	35.7	D
50	M	S5	22			15M	48.9	C	10	4.8	35.9	AD
67	M	S8	11		LLR		39	A	6	5	47.9	A
67	F	S8-4,S5,S6	32	Open			34.6	A	6	7.2	58.7	D
40	M	S6	20			60M	52.5	B	7	6	75.6	D
61	M	S5	15				70.8	A	5	11.9	127.8	A

S: segment, HALS: hand-assisted laparoscopic surgery, LT: liver transplantation, CP: Child-Pugh classification and score, EVL: patients who underwent endoscopic varices ligation before LLR, A: alive, D: dead of hepatocellular carcinoma or liver disease, AD: dead of the other cause.

Table 3. Parameters of liver function in the patient groups of those who survived more than 24 months (A*) and who died of HCC or liver disease within 24 months (D)

Platelet counts, $\times 10^4/\mu L$		
Group	A (n = 10)	D** (n = 6)
Mean+/-SD	10.740+/-9.426	5.567+/-1.516
Unpaired t two-tailed P-value = 0.2093		

CP score		
Group	A (n = 10)	D (n = 7)
Mean+/-SD	6.50+/-1.35	8.14+/-1.21
Unpaired t two-tailed P-value = 0.0216#		

ICGR15, %		
Group	A (n = 10)	D (n = 7)
Mean+/-SD	48.420+/-14.600	44.786+/-10.560
Unpaired t two-tailed P-value = 0.5828		

*1 patient who underwent liver transplantation at 15 months after LR was excluded from group A; **1 patient after splenectomy was excluded from group D; # statistically different. CP: Child-Pugh classification score; HCC: Hepatocellular carcinoma; ICGR15: Indocyanine green retention rate at 15 min.

Excluding the 1 patient whose follow-up period is less than 24 mo and the 1 patient who underwent LT at 15 months after LLR, 7 patients died of HCC or liver disease within 24 months after LLR (D group). When the D patients were compared to the group of 10 patients who survived more than 24 months (A group), there are significant difference in CP scores between the groups (Table 3). The values of ICGR15 are similar in the A and D groups. All of the D patients, but only 3 of the 11 A patients, had esophageal varices before surgery. All of the A patients, excluding the patients with LT at 15 months, had 50,000 or more blood platelet counts, and 5 out of 7 D patients had below 60,000.

It is thought that ICGR15 above 30%-40% is out of their reliable range and not well-correlated with actual liver function. Thus, it may not be suitable for the liver functional selection criteria of surface small LLR, even though it is very useful and simple criteria for judging how much liver volume can be resected in the range below 30%-40%. Although the difficult judgements for the objective presences of ascites and encephalopathy should be needed, CP score is a promising candidate for selection indicator of surface small LLR, correlating well to our indication criteria, patient's performance status, and prognosis after the surgery. Portal hypertension [76], indicated by the presence of esophageal varices and low platelet counts, should be also counted in the selection of surface small LLR.

Most reported cases of repeat LLR underwent minor resection for HCC patients with CLD, as mentioned above. The impact of alterations to hepatic parenchyma and intrahepatic structural anatomy from the previous LR could be relatively small in such cases. However, in our experience of 33 repeat and 12 three or more-time repeat LLRs, three patients who underwent anatomical resection or resections exposing major vessels (including S8 segmentectomy after 4-times LLR [77]) after previous anatomical resection developed postoperative bile leakage and more than 30 days postoperative hospital stay. Since anatomical alterations and surrounding scars and/or adhesion of hilar and intrahepatic vessel structures should have big impacts on anatomical resection or resections exposing major vessels as repeat LLR after previous anatomical resection, further experiences and evaluations of such repeat LLR are needed.

CONCLUSION

The characteristics mentioned above indicate that LLR may be superior to OLR under certain conditions. The LLR could also be an optional bridging therapy to LT for certain HCC patients with severe CLD [31]. The recent development of LLR and accumulation of experience could lead to an expansion of the indication for LLR [45]. Although the number of studies reported has been small and comprising various settings, we believe that the features of LLR that have come to light will lead to expanding the indications for LR to HCC patients with background CLD, particularly in the settings of severe CLD, repeat LR and bridging to LT.

REFERENCES

[1] Capussotti L, Ferrero A, Viganò L, Polastri R, Tabone M. Liver resection for HCC with cirrhosis: surgical perspectives out of EASL/AASLD guidelines. *Eur J Surg Oncol.* 2009;35:11-15. [PMID: 17689043 DOI: 10.1016/j.ejso.2007.06.005].

[2] Hwang S, Lee SG, Belghiti J. Liver transplantation for HCC: its role: Eastern and Western perspectives. *J Hepatobiliary Pancreat Sci.* 2010;17:443-448. [PMID: 19885638 DOI: 10.1007/s00534-009-0241-0].

[3] Lau WY, Leung TW, Yu SC, Ho SK. Percutaneous local ablative therapy for hepatocellular carcinoma: a review and look into the future. *Ann Surg.* 2003;237:171-179. [PMID: 12560774 DOI: 10. 1097/01.SLA.0000048443.71734.BF].

[4] Mazzaferro V1, Regalia E, Doci R, Andreola S, Pulvirenti A, Bozzetti F, Montalto F, Ammatuna M, Morabito A, Gennari L. Liver transplantation for the treatment of small hepatocellular carcinomas in patients with cirrhosis. *N Engl J Med.* 1996;334:693-699. [PMID: 8594428 DOI: 10.1056/NEJM199603143341104].

[5] Ryder SD. Guidelines for the diagnosis and treatment of hepatocellular carcinoma (HCC) in adults. *Gut.* 2003;52(Suppl 3):iii1-8. [PMID: 12692148 PMCID: PMC1867754].

[6] Morise Z, Kawabe N, Tomishige H, Nagata H, Kawase J, Arakawa S, Yoshida R, Isetani M. Recent advances in the surgical treatment of hepatocellular carcinoma. *World J Gastroenterol.* 2014;20 (39): 14381-92. [PMID: 25339825 DOI: 10.3748/wjg.v20.i39.14381.].

[7] Llovet JM, Fuster J, Bruix J. The Barcelona approach: diagnosis, staging, and treatment of hepatocellular carcinoma. *Liver Transpl.* 2004;10:S115–S120. [PMID: 14762851 DOI: 10.1002/lt.20034].

[8] Llovet JM, Fuster J, Bruix J. Intention-to-treat analysis of surgical treatment for early hepatocellular carcinoma: resection versus transplantation. *Hepatology* 1999;30:1434–1440. [PMID: 10573522 DOI: 10.1002/hep.510300629].

[9] Cucchetti A, Vitale A, Gaudio MD, Pinna AD. Harm and benefits of primary liver resection and salvage transplantation for hepatocellular carcinoma. *Am J Transplant* 2010; 10: 619-627. [PMID: 20121741 DOI: 10.1111/j.1600-6143.2009.02984.x].

[10] Yao FY, Ferrell L, Bass NM, Watson JJ, Bacchetti P, Venook A, Ascher NL, Roberts JP. Liver transplantation for hepatocellular carcinoma: Expansion of the tumor size limits does not adversely impact survival. *Hepatology* 2001; 33: 1394-1403. [PMID: 11391528 DOI: 10.1053/jhep.2001.24563].

[11] Fujiki M, Takada Y, Ogura Y, Oike F, Kaido T, Teramukai S, Uemoto S. Significance of des-gamma-carboxy prothrombin in selection criteria for living donor liver transplantation for hepatocellular carcinoma. *Am J Transplant* 2009; 9(10): 2362-71. [PMID: 19656125 DOI: 10.1111/j.1600-6143.2009.02783.x].

[12] Bruix J, Reig M, Sherman M. Evidence-based diagnosis, staging, and treatment of patients with hepatocellular carcinoma. *Gastroenterology* 2016;150:836–853. [PMID: 26795574 DOI: 10.1053/j.gastro.2015.12.041].

[13] Bruix J, Castells A, Bosch J, Feu F, Fuster J, Garcia-Pagan J, Visa J, Bru C, Rodes J. Surgical resection of hepatocellular carcinoma in cirrhotic patients: prognostic value of preoperative portal pressure. *Gastroenterology.* 1996;111:1018-22. [PMID: 8831597 DOI:10.1016/ S0016-5085(96)70070-7].

[14] Hoeper MM, Krowka MJ, Strassburg CP. Portopulmonary hypertension and hepatopulmonary syndrome. *Lancet.* 2004;363 (9419):1461-1468. [PMID: 15121411 DOI: 10.1016/S0140-6736 (04)16107-2].

[15] Ziser A, Plevak DJ, Wiesner RH, Rakela J, Offord KP, Brown DL. Morbidity and mortality in cirrhotic patients undergoing anesthesia and surgery. *Anesthesiology*. 1999;90:42-53. [PMID: 9915311].

[16] Mansour A, Watson W, Shayani V, Pickleman J. Abdominal operations in patients with cirrhosis: still a major surgical challenge. *Surgery*. 1997;122:730-735. [PMID: 9347849].

[17] Belghiti J, Hiramatsu K, Benoist S, Massault P, Sauvanet A, Farges O. Seven hundred forty-seven hepatectomies in the 1990s: an update to evaluate the actual risk of liver resection. *J Am Coll Surg*. 2000;191:38-46. [PMID: 10898182].

[18] Lai EC, Fan ST, Lo CM, Chu KM, Liu CL, Wong J. Hepatic resection for hepatocellular carcinoma. An audit of 343 patients. *Ann Surg*. 1995;221:291-298. [PMID: 7717783 PMCID: PMC1234572].

[19] Rahbari NN, Mehrabi A, Mollberg NM, Muller SA, Koch M, Buchler MW, Weitz J. Hepatocellular carcinoma: current management and perspectives for the future. *Ann Surg* 2011; 253: 453-469. [PMID: 21263310 DOI: 10.1097/SLA.0b013e31820d944f].

[20] Torzilli G, Belghiti J, Kokudo N, Takayama T, Capussotti L, Nuzzo G, Vauthey JN, Choti MA, De Santibanes E, Donadon M, Morenghi E, Makuuchi M. A snapshot of the effective indications and results of surgery for hepatocellular carcinoma in tertiary referral centers: is it adherent to the EASL/AASLD recommendations?: an observational study of the HCC East-West study group. *Ann Surg*. 2013;257:929-37. [PMID: 23426336 DOI: 10.1097/SLA.0b013e31828329b8].

[21] El-Serag HB, Marrero JA, Rudolph L, Reddy KR. Diagnosis and treatment of hepatocellular carcinoma. *Gastroenterology* 2008; 134: 1752-1763. [PMID: 18471552 DOI: 10.1053/j.gastro.2008.02.090].

[22] Forner A, Reig ME, de Lope CR, Bruix J. Current strategy for staging and treatment: the BCLC update and future prospects. *Semin Liver Dis* 2010; 30: 61-74. [PMID: 20175034 DOI: 10.1055/s-0030-1247133].

[23] World Consensus Conference on Laparoscopic Surgery. The international position on laparoscopic liver surgery: The Louisville

Statement, 2008. *Ann Surg* 2009; 250(5): 825-30. [PMID: 19916210 DOI: 10.1097/SLA.0b013e3181b3b2d8].

[24] Wakabayashi G, Cherqui D, Geller DA, Buell JF, Kaneko H, Han HS, Asbun H, O'Rourke N, Tanabe M, Koffron AJ, Tsung A, Soubrane O, Machado MA, Gayet B, Troisi RI, Pessaux P, Van Dam RM, Scatton O, Abu Hilal M, Belli G, Kwon CH, Edwin B, Choi GH, Aldrighetti LA, Cai X, Cleary S, Chen KH, Schön MR, Sugioka A, Tang CN, Herman P, Pekolj J, Chen XP, Dagher I, Jarnagin W, Yamamoto M, Strong R, Jagannath P, Lo CM, Clavien PA, Kokudo N, Barkun J, Strasberg SM. Recommendations for laparoscopic liver resection: a report from the second international consensus conference held in Morioka. *Ann Surg*. 2015;261:619-29. [PMID: 25742461 DOI: 10.1097/SLA.0000000000001184].

[25] Reich H, McGlynn F, DeCaprio J, Budin R. Laparoscopic excision of benign liver lesions. *Obstet Gynecol* 1991; 78 (5 Pt 2): 956-958. [PMID: 1833688].

[26] Katkhouda N, Fabiani P, Benizri E, Mouiel J. Laser resection of a liver hydatid cyst under videolaparoscopy. *Br J Surg*. 1992; 79(6): 560-1. [PMID: 1535261].

[27] Gagner M, Rheault M, Dubuc J. Laparoscopic partial hepatectomy for liver tumor. *Surg Endosc* 1992; 6: 97-98. (abstract).

[28] Viganò L, Tayar C, Laurent A, Cherqui D. Laparoscopic liver resection: a systematic review. *J Hepatobiliary Pancreat Surg* 2009; 16(4): 410-21. [PMID: 19495556 DOI: 10.1007/s00534-009-0120-8].

[29] Mirnezami R, Mirnezami AH, Chandrakumaran K, Abu Hilal M, Pearce NW, Primrose JN, Sutcliffe RP. Short- and long-term outcomes after laparoscopic and open hepatic resection: systematic review and meta-analysis. *HPB* 2011; 13(5): 295–308. [PMID: 21492329 DOI: 10.1111/j.1477-2574.2011.00295.x].

[30] Belli G, Fantini C, Belli A, Limongelli P. Laparoscopic liver resection for hepatocellular carcinoma in cirrhosis: long term outcomes. *Dig Surg* 2011; 28: 134-140. [PMID: 21540599 DOI: 10.1159/000323824].

[31] Morise Z, Kawabe N, Kawase J, Tomishige H, Nagata H, Ohshima H, Arakawa S, Yoshida R, Isetani M. Pure laparoscopic hepatectomy for hepatocellular carcinoma with chronic liver disease. *World J Hepatol* 2013 Sep 27; 5(9): 487-495. [PMID: 24073300].

[32] Tranchart H, Di Giuro G, Lainas P, Roudie J, Agostini H, Franco D, Dagher I. Laparoscopic resection for hepatocellular carcinoma: a matched-pair comparative study. *Surg Endosc* 2010; 24(5): 1170-6. [PMID: 19915908 DOI: 10.1007/s00464-009-0745-3].

[33] Morise Z, Ciria R, Cherqui D, Chen KH, Belli G, Wakabayashi G. Can we expand the indications for laparoscopic liver resection? A systematic review and meta-analysis of laparoscopic liver resection for patients with hepatocellular carcinoma and chronic liver disease. J Hepatobiliary *Pancreat Sci.* 2015;22:342–352. [PMID: 25663288 DOI: 10.1002/jhbp.215].

[34] Tomishige H, Morise Z, Kawabe N, Nagata H, Ohshima H, Kawase J, Arakawa S, Yoshida R, Isetani M. Caudal approach to pure laparoscopic posterior sectionectomy under the laparoscopy-specific view. *World J Gastrointest Surg* 2013;5:173-7. PMID: 23977419 DOI: 10.4240/wjgs.v5.i6.173.

[35] Soubrane O, Schwarz L, Cauchy F, Cauchy F, Perotto LO, Brustia R, et al. A conceptual technique for laparoscopic right hepatectomy based on facts and oncologic principles: the caudal approach. *Ann Surg*. 2015;261:1226-31. PMID: 24854453 DOI: 10.1097/SLA.000 0000000000737.

[36] Wakabayashi G, Cherqui D, Geller DA, Han HS, Kaneko H, Buell JF. Laparoscopic hepatectomy is theoretically better than open hepatectomy: preparing for the 2nd International Consensus Conference on Laparoscopic Liver Resection. *J Hepatobiliary Pancreat Sci.* 2014;21:723-731. PMID: 25130985 DOI: 10.1002/ jhbp.139.

[37] Morise Z. Laparoscopic liver resection for posterosuperior tumors using caudal approach and postural changes: A new technical approach. *World J Gastroenterol.* 2016;22:10267-10274. PMID: 28058008 DOI: 10.3748/wjg.v22.i47.10267.

[38] Morise Z, Sugioka A, Kawabe N, Umemoto S, Nagata H, Ohshima H, Kawase J, Arakawa S, Yoshida R. Pure laparoscopic hepatectomy for hepatocellular carcinoma patients with severe liver cirrhosis. *Asian J Endosc Surg* 2011; 4(3): 143-6. [PMID: 22776279 DOI: 10.1111/j.1758-5910.2011.00081.x].

[39] Petrowsky H, Gonen M, Jarnagin W, Lorenz M, DeMatteo R, Heinrich S, Encke A, Blumgart L, Fong Y. Second liver resections are safe and effective treatment for recurrent hepatic metastases from colorectal cancer: a bi-institutional analysis. *Ann Surg* 2002; 235: 863-871 PMID: 12035044 DOI: 10.1097/00000658-200206000-00015.

[40] Wanebo HJ, Chu QD, Avradopoulos KA, Vezeridis MP. Current perspectives on repeat hepatic resection for colorectal carcinoma: a review. *Surgery* 1996; 119: 361-371 PMID: 8643998 DOI: 10.1016/S0039-6060(96)80133-4.

[41] Morise Z, Sugioka A, Fujita J, Hoshimoto S, Kato T, Hasumi A, Suda T, Negi H, Hattori Y, Sato H, Maeda K. Does repeated surgery improve the prognosis of colorectal liver metastases? *J Gastrointest Surg.* 2006 Jan;10(1):6-11. PMID: 16368485 DOI: 10.1016/j.gassur.2005.09.006.

[42] Itamoto T, Nakahara H, Amano H, Kohashi T, Ohdan H, Tashiro H, Asahara T. Repeat hepatectomy for recurrent hepatocellular carcinoma. *Surgery* 2007; 141: 589-597 PMID: 17462458 DOI: 10.1016/j.surg.2006.12.014.

[43] Nguyen KT, Gamblin TC, Geller DA. World review of laparoscopic liver resection-2,804 patients. *Ann Surg* 2009; 250: 831-841 PMID: 19801936 DOI: 10.1097/SLA.0b013e3181b0c4df.

[44] Buell JF, Thomas MT, Rudich S, Marvin M, Nagubandi R, Ravindra KV, Brock G, McMasters KM. Experience with more than 500 minimally invasive hepatic procedures. *Ann Surg* 2008; 248: 475-486 PMID: 18791368.

[45] Morise Z, Wakabayashi G. First quarter century of laparoscopic liver resection. *World J Gastroenterol.* 2017;23(20):3581-3588. PMID: 28611511 DOI: 10.3748/wjg.v23.i20.3581.

[46] Beck DE, Ferguson MA, Opelka FG, Fleshman JW, Gervaz P, Wexner SD. Effect of previous surgery on abdominal opening time. *Dis Colon Rectum* 2000; 43: 1749-1753 PMID: 11156462 DOI: 10.1007/BF02236862.

[47] Karayiannakis AJ, Polychronidis A, Perente S, Botaitis S, Simopoulos C. Laparoscopic cholecystectomy in patients with previous upper or lower abdominal surgery. *Surg Endosc* 2004; 18: 97-101 PMID: 14569455 DOI: 10.1007/ s00464-003-9001-4.

[48] Wiebke EA, Pruitt AL, Howard TJ, Jacobson LE, Broadie TA, Goulet RJ, Canal DF. Conversion of laparoscopic to open cholecystectomy. An analysis of risk factors. *Surg Endosc* 1996; 10: 742-745 PMID: 8662431 DOI: 10.1007/BF00193048.

[49] Wu JM, Lin HF, Chen KH, Tseng LM, Tsai MS, Huang SH. Impact of previous abdominal surgery on laparoscopic appendectomy for acute appendicitis. *Surg Endosc* 2007; 21: 570-573 PMID: 17103279 DOI: 10.1007/s00464-006-9027-5.

[50] Law WL, Lee YM, Chu KW. Previous abdominal operations do not affect the outcomes of laparoscopic colorectal surgery. *Surg Endosc* 2005; 19: 326-330 PMID: 15624064 DOI: 10.1007/ s00464-004-8114-8.

[51] Nunobe S, Hiki N, Fukunaga T, Tokunaga M, Ohyama S, Seto Y, Yamaguchi T. Previous laparotomy is not a contraindication to laparoscopy-assisted gastrectomy for early gastric cancer. *World J Surg* 2008; 32: 1466-1472 PMID: 18340481 DOI: 10.1007/s00268-008-9542-8.

[52] Szomstein S, Lo Menzo E, Simpfendorfer C, Zundel N, Rosenthal RJ. Laparoscopic lysis of adhesions. *World J Surg* 2006; 30: 535-540 PMID: 16555020 DOI: 10.1007/ s00268-005-7778-0.

[53] Ome Y, Hashida K, Yokota M, Nagahisa Y, Yamaguchi K, Okabe M, Kawamoto K. The feasibility and efficacy of pure laparoscopic repeat hepatectomy. *Surg Endosc.* 2018;[Epub ahead of print]. PMID: 29344784 DOI: 10.1007/s00464-018-6066-7.

[54] Noda T, Eguchi H, Wada H, Iwagami Y, Yamada D, Asaoka T, Gotoh K, Kawamoto K, Takeda Y, Tanemura M, Umeshita K, Doki

Y, Mori M. Short-term surgical outcomes of minimally invasive repeat hepatectomy for recurrent liver cancer. *Surg Endosc.* 2018;32(1):46-52. PMID: 28639044 DOI: 10.1007/s00464-017-5632-8.

[55] Belli G, Cioffi L, Fantini C, D'Agostino A, Russo G, Limongelli P, Belli A. Laparoscopic redo surgery for recurrent hepatocellular carcinoma in cirrhotic patients: feasibility, safety, and results. *Surg Endosc.* 2009;23:1807-11. PMID: 19277781 DOI: 10.1007/s00464-009-0344-3.

[56] Nguyen KT, Laurent A, Dagher I, Geller DA, Steel J, Thomas MT, Marvin M, Ravindra KV, Mejia A, Lainas P, Franco D, Cherqui D, Buell JF, Gamblin TC. Minimally invasive liver resection for metastatic colorectal cancer: a multi-institutional, international report of safety, feasibility, and early outcomes. *Ann Surg.* 2009;250:842-8. PMID: 19806058 DOI: 10.1097/SLA.0b013e3181bc789c.

[57] Ahn KS, Han HS, Yoon YS, Cho JY, Kim JH. Laparoscopic liver resection in patients with a history of upper abdominal surgery. *World J Surg.* 2011;35:1333-9. PMID: 21452069 DOI: 10.1007/s00 268-011-1073-z.

[58] Shafaee Z, Kazaryan AM, Marvin MR, Cannon R, Buell JF, Edwin B, Gayet B. Is laparoscopic repeat hepatectomy feasible? A tri-institutional analysis. *J Am Coll Surg.* 2011;212:171-9. PMID: 21276531 DOI: 10.1016/j.jamcollsurg.2010.10.012.

[59] Hu M, Zhao G, Xu D, Liu R. Laparoscopic repeat resection of recurrent hepatocellular carcinoma. *World J Surg.* 2011;35:648-55. PMID: 21184074 DOI: 10.1007/s00268-010-0919-0.

[60] Cannon RM, Brock GN, Marvin MR, Buell JF. Laparoscopic liver resection: an examination of our first 300 patients. *J Am Coll Surg.* 2011;213:501-7. PMID: 21624840 DOI: 10.1016/j.jamcollsurg. 2011.04.032.

[61] Tsuchiya M, Otsuka Y, Maeda T, Ishii J, Tamura A, Kaneko H. Efficacy of laparoscopic surgery for recurrent hepatocellular carcinoma. *Hepatogastroenterology.* 2012;59:1333-7. PMID: 2259 1625 DOI: 10.5754/hge12302.

[62] Kanazawa A, Tsukamoto T, Shimizu S, Kodai S, Yamamoto S, Yamazoe S, Ohira G, Nakajima T. Laparoscopic liver resection for treating recurrent hepatocellular carcinoma. *J Hepatobiliary Pancreat* Sci. 2013;20:512-7. PMID: 23404252 DOI: 10.1007/s00534-012-0592-9.

[63] Montalti R, Berardi G, Laurent S, Sebastiani S, Ferdinande L, Libbrecht LJ, Smeets P, Brescia A, Rogiers X, de Hemptinne B, Geboes K, Troisi RI. Laparoscopic liver resection compared to open approach in patients with colorectal liver metastases improves further respectability: Oncological outcomes of a case-control matched-pairs analysis. *Eur J Surg Oncol.* 2014;40:536-44. PMID: 24555996 DOI: 10.1016/j.ejso.2014.01.005.

[64] Isetani M, Morise Z, Kawabe N, Tomishige H, Nagata H, Kawase J, Arakawa S. Pure laparoscopic hepatectomy as repeat surgery and repeat hepatectomy. *World J Gastroenterol.* 2015;21:961-8. PMID: 25624731 DOI: 10.3748/wjg.v21.i3.961.

[65] Shelat VG1, Serin K, Samim M, Besselink MG, Al Saati H, Gioia PD, Pearce NW, Abu Hilal M. Outcomes of repeat laparoscopic liver resection compared to the primary resection. *World J Surg.* 2014; 38:3175-80. PMID: 25138071 DOI: 10.1007/s00268-014-2728-3.

[66] Goh BKP, Teo JY, Chan CY, Lee SY, Cheow PC, Chung AYF. Laparoscopic repeat liver resection for recurrent hepatocellular carcinoma. *ANZ J Surg.* 2017;87(10):E143-E146. PMID: 27117542 DOI: 10.1111/ans.13628.

[67] Hallet J, Sa Cunha A, Cherqui D, Gayet B, Goéré D, Bachellier P, Laurent A, Fuks D, Navarro F, Pessaux P; French Colorectal Liver Metastases Working Group, Association Française de Chirurgie. Laparoscopic Compared to Open Repeat Hepatectomy for Colorectal Liver Metastases: a Multi-institutional Propensity-Matched Analysis of Short- and Long-Term Outcomes. *World J Surg.* 2017; 41 (12):3189-3198. PMID: 28717911 DOI: 10.1007/s00268-017-4119-z.

[68] Chan AC, Poon RT, Chok KS, Cheung TT, Chan SC, Lo CM. Feasibility of laparoscopic re-resection for patients with recurrent

hepatocellular carcinoma. *World J Surg*. 2014;38(5):1141-6. PMID: 24305932 DOI: 10.1007/s00268-013-2380-3.

[69] Bruix J, Sherman M Management of hepatocellular carcinoma: An update. *Hepatology*. 2011; 53: 1020–1022. [PMID: 21374666 DOI: 10.1002/hep.24199].

[70] Kudo M, Izumi N, Kokudo N, Matsui O, Sakamoto M, Nakashima O, Kojiro M, Makuuchi M; HCC Expert Panel of Japan Society of Hepatology. Management of hepatocellular carcinoma in Japan: Consensus-Based Clinical Practice Guidelines proposed by the Japan Society of Hepatology (JSH) 2010 updated version. *Dig Dis*. 2011;29(3):339-64. [PMID: 21829027 DOI: 10.1159/000327577].

[71] Pugh RN, Murray-Lyon IM, Dawson JL, Pietroni MC, Williams R. Transection of the oesophagus for bleeding oesophageal varices. *Br J Surg*. 1973 Aug;60(8):646-9. No abstract available. [PMID: 4541913].

[72] Omagari K, Ohba K, Kadokawa Y, Hazama H, Masuda J, Kinoshita H, Matsuo I, Ohnita K, Mizuta Y, Hayashida K, Kohno S. Comparison of the grade evaluated by "Liver damage" of Liver Cancer Study Group of Japan and Child-Pugh classification in patients with hepatocellular carcinoma. *Hepatol Res*. 2006;34:266-72. [PMID: 16460997 DOI: 10.1016/j.hepres.2005.05.010].

[73] Lau H, Man K, Fan ST, Yu WC, Lo CM, Wong J. Evaluation of preoperative hepatic function in patients with hepatocellular carcinoma undergoing hepatectomy. *Br J Surg*. 1997;84:1255-9. [PMID: 9313707].

[74] Makuuchi M, Kosuge T, Takayama T, Yamazaki S, Kakazu T, Miyagawa S, Kawasaki S. Surgery for small liver cancers. *Semin Surg Oncol*. 1993;9:298-304. [PMID: 8210909].

[75] Nonami T, Nakao A, Kurokawa T, Inagaki H, Matsushita Y, Sakamoto J, Takagi H. Blood loss and ICG clearance as best prognostic markers of post-hepatectomy liver failure. *Hepato-gastroenterology*. 1999;46:1669-72. [PMID: 10430318].

[76] Molina V, Sampson-Dávila J, Ferrer J, Fondevila C, Díaz Del Gobbo R, Calatayud D, Bruix J, García-Valdecasas JC, Fuster J. Benefits of

laparoscopic liver resection in patients with hepatocellular carcinoma and portal hypertension: a case-matched study. *Surg Endosc*. 2017 Dec 7. [Epub ahead of print] [PMID: 29218665 DOI: 10.1007/s00464-017-5930-1].

[77] Morise Z, Isetani M, Kawabe N, Tomishige H, Nagata H, Arakawa S, Ikeda M, Kamio K. Case report of the fourth laparoscopic liver resection and review of repeat laparoscopic resection for recurrent hepatocellular carcinoma in cirrhotic liver. *Hepatoma Res* 2016;2:253-8. DOI: 10.20517/2394-5079.2016.09.

In: Handbook of Surgical Procedures
Editor: Heather Gilbert
ISBN: 978-1-53614-580-9

Chapter 3

MEDICAL AND SURGICAL ADVANCES IN BRONCHOSCOPY

Jack A Kastelik*[1,*], *MD, Mahmoud Loubani*[2], *MD, Kate Dixon*[3], *BA and Keyvan Moghissi*[3], *MD

[1]Department of Academic Respiratory Medicine
University of Hull, Hull York Medical School
Castle Hill Hospital Castle Road, Cottingham
East Yorkshire, UK
[2]Department of Cardiothoracic Surgery
University of Hull, Hull York Medical School
Castle Hill Hospital, Castle Road, Cottingham
East Yorkshire, UK
[3]Yorkshire Laser Centre
Goole and District Hospital, Woodlands Avenue,
Goole, East Yorkshire, US

[*] Corresponding Author Email: Dr JA Kastelik, Email: jack.kastelik@hey.nhs.uk.

ABSTRACT

Bronchoscopy has become an important procedure, which is performed for diagnostic and therapeutic purposes. There has been very important expansion in the application of bronchoscopy due to technological developments. Bronchoscopic techniques have acquired use as diagnostic procedures in the context of infection or malignancy. Over recent years, procedures such as endobronchial ultrasound have become widely used. Similarly, new technologies such as navigational bronchoscopy are becoming more commonly used. In addition, bronchoscopy has extended its application into interventional procedures. For example, in the context of Chronic Obstructive Pulmonary Disease, bronchoscopic insertion of endobrochial valves has become widely used. Bronchoscopy also can be used for photodynamic therapy in the context of lung cancer. In this chapter the medical and surgical advances in bronchoscopy will be described.

Keywords: bronchoscopy, endobronchial valves, endobronchial ultrasound, photodynamic therapy

INTRODUCTION

Bronchoscopy has become an important procedure, which is performed for diagnostic and therapeutic purposes. It is a common procedure with over 500,000 bronchoscopies being performed in the USA each year (Ernst, Silvestri, and Johnstone 2003, Silvestri et al. 2012). Due to technological developments, as well as improvements in imaging bronchoscopy, techniques have become more complex. The first bronchoscopy was performed by Gustav Killian in 1897 to remove a foreign body from the patient's main bronchus (Batra and Yarmus 2018). Subsequently, the rigid bronchoscope became an important tool for examination of the proximal bronchi. The main limitations of rigid bronchoscopy include the requirements for general anaesthesia and the fact that it only allows visualization of the carina and main bronchi (Annigeri and Patil 2017). In 1967 Shigeto Ikeda introduced flexible bronchoscopy, which allowed for visualization beyond the main bronchi. Flexible bronchoscopy has other advantages compared with rigid bronchoscopy. The procedure is performed under an awake sedation, seldom requiring general anaesthesia. The technique is easier to master, compared to rigid bronchoscopy, which may be technically more difficult. Over recent years, due to technological developments, there have been new techniques introduced such as auto-fluorescence bronchoscopy, endobronchial ultrasound, electromagnetic navigational bronchoscopy, photodynamic therapy bronchoscopy and endobronchial valves (Mehta et al. 2018)

FLEXIBLE FIBREOPTIC BRONCHOSCOPY

Flexible fibreoptic bronchoscopes have glass fibres, which allow for light to be transported from the light source to the distal part of the scope, delivering images from the end of the scope to a high definition screen (Du Rand et al. 2013). The flexible fibreoptic bronchoscope has instrumentation and suctioning channels, therefore it allows for both the examination of the bronchial tree and introduction of instruments such bronchial brushes or bronchial biopsy forceps. Therapeutic scopes have a larger instrument channel allowing for the introduction of instruments which can be used for diagnostic and therapeutic purposes (Du Rand et al. 2011).

Fiberoptic bronchoscopy is usually undertaken in the endoscopy suite or operating theatre, supported by staff capable of preparing the equipment, managing the collected samples and caring for sedated patients. The operator needs to be skilled in the administration of awake sedation, potential indications or contraindications and complications of the procedure, as well as having extensive knowledge of bronchial anatomy and pathology (Wahidi et al. 2011). The learning of bronchoscopy skills is a complex process (Rayl, Pittman, and Shuster 1988, Silvestri et al. 2012). However, the historical apprenticeship type of learning of bronchoscopy skills is gradually changing with the wider application of simulation technology (Kvale and Mehta 2001, Silvestri 2008). This approach, based on simulation training of the procedural skills in the laboratory, reduces the stress of the learning of complex procedures, when compared to learning in clinical settings; it can used in conjunction with lectures or web based teaching (Blum, Powers, and Sundaresan 2004, Davoudi and Colt 2009, Haponik et al. 2000, Torrington 2000).

Fiberoptic bronchoscopy can incorporate auto-fluorescence, which has higher sensitivity to detect early or precancerous changes, though it is mainly used for diagnostic purposes. Therefore, procedures such as bronchial washing, bronchial brushing and bronchial or trans-bronchial biopsies are the most common procedures undertaken during bronchoscopy (Du Rand et al. 2013). One of the other important aspects of fiberoptic bronchoscopy includes bronchial secretion clearance, which may be of particular use in patients on mechanical ventilation. From the diagnostic aspect, perhaps the most common application of fiberoptic bronchoscopy is in the diagnosis of lung cancer. This is of particular importance in patients with visible endobronchial tumours which can be biopsied during the procedure; additionally, it can be used pre operatively to plan surgery. Moreover, fiberoptic bronchoscopy performed by a skilled operator can be used for retrieval of a foreign body, although a rigid bronchoscopy may be more appropriate (Du Rand et al. 2011). The rigid bronchoscope may allow better access for the removal of the foreign body, controlling of bleeding, ability to introduce larger instruments and, as it is performed under general anaesthesia, better oxygenation control as well as more appropriate access to interventional procedures if required.

PHOTODYNAMIC THERAPY

Photodynamic therapy (PDT) is a treatment which comprises of a chemical photosensitizer, a matching wavelength of light, usually generated by laser, and oxygen, which is present in all living tissues. The interaction between light and photosensitizer, in the presence of oxygen, generates singlet oxygen and other cytotoxic species leading to cell death (Allison and Moghissi 2013). For central lung cancer PDT is carried out bronchoscopically, as a two-step procedure (Moghissi and Dixon 2008,

2003, Okunaka and Kato 2002, Ikeda et al. 2011). The first step, pre-sensitization, involves intravenous administration of photosensitizer, which is distributed throughout the body; a higher concentration will be retained within the cancer compared with normal, surrounding tissues. The second step is illumination, during which the pre-sensitized cancer tissue in the airway is exposed to an appropriate laser light transmitted via an optical fiber, which is passed through the bronchoscope. The cancer tissue containing photosensitizer, in the presence of oxygen, is activated by the laser light, prompting destruction of cancerous tissue. The pre-requisite for bronchoscopic PDT is the presence of an endo-luminal, biopsy proven, malignant tumour in the airway, following standard investigations and staging procedures. Standard treatment for malignant broncho-pulmonary tumours consists of surgery, radiotherapy and chemotherapy. However, a number of other "non-standard" options have recently become available, all of which are basically local therapies. PDT is one such option with a number of important attributes. PDT is the only method amongst non-standard therapies, which specifically targets cancer with the exclusion of healthy surrounding tissue.

Bronchoscopic PDT in lung cancer can be used in the context of an early stage central endobronchial cancer with the aim of 'curative intent' (Ikeda et al. 2011, Moghissi et al. 2007). Also, PDT can be considered in locally advanced inoperable endobronchial cancer (Moghissi et al. 2007, Okunaka and Kato 2002). Here, the aim is to open up a lobar or main stem bronchus, which is blocked by cancer, thus allowing pulmonary ventilation. There is an increasing tendency to use PDT in such cases within a multi modal protocol (Ikeda et al. 2011). Another application of PDT is in metachronous, endobronchial tumours of the residual lung after previous resection for local bronchial stump recurrence as an induction therapy prior to surgery and for rare bronchial tumours, such as carcinoid and adenoid cystic carcinoma (Moghissi et al. 2007, Moghissi and Dixon 2003, Ross et al. 2006, Akopov et al. 2017, Moghissi and Dixon 2017). However, in practice all cases fall within endobronchial malignancies confined to bronchial mucosa with no parenchymal lesion and without nodal or distant metastases. PDT can be offered with curative intent for locally advanced cancers, which are bulky endobronchial tumours with no distant metastases but with atelectasis. In these, PDT offers palliation with survival benefit in some.

Prior to bronchoscopic PDT, an informed consent should include information on photosensitivity skin reaction to direct or indirect sunlight exposure. Bronchoscopic assessment should aim to delineate the extent and topography of tumour using white light and auto fluorescence bronchoscopy. Currently, Photofrin (Porfimer Sodium) is the photo-sensitizer of choice. The interval between drug administration and treatment allows wide distribution in the body and retention predominantly in cancer tissues. There are two methods available for illumination. During the first method, which is performed under general anesthesia, the rigid bronchoscope is initially inserted, through which the flexible fiberoptic bronchoscope is subsequently introduced. Exposure to light of the pre-sensitized tissue is undertaken via an optical fiber; this is passed through the biopsy channel of the flexible fiberoptic bronchoscope. The second method uses a flexible fiberoptic bronchoscope under awake sedation and local anesthesia. The optical fiber is passed through the biopsy channel of the flexible fiberoptic bronchoscope, directing the laser light to the target. Bronchoscopic PDT under general anaesthesia is the preferred method, except when this is not possible or rejected by the patient, as it allows for better airway protection, reduces coughing and improves patient comfort. Current literature suggests that PDT in the context of an early lung cancer may achieve long survival in between 60 -70% of cases (Ikeda et al. 2011, Okunaka and Kato 2002). In locally advanced cases PDT offers good palliation with improved pulmonary function and survival benefit in some cases (Moghissi et al. 2007, Moghissi et al. 1999). It is relevant to point out that PDT can be used with standard treatments, notably chemo-radiation; it is a treatment, which can be repeated. The only problem can be photosensitivity skin reaction over a variable duration, according to the photosensitizer employed, hence the need for effective patient counseling.

Endobronchial Valves

Patients with Chronic Obstructive Pulmonary Disease (COPD) have increased lung compliance and airway resistance, due to small airway obstruction leading to air trapping, resulting in the increase in total lung capacity (TLC) and residual volume (RV) leading to hyperinflation (Herth et al. 2016). During exercise the respiratory rate is increased which, in turn, leads to a shorter time for lung emptying; this, in turn, increases end expiratory lung volume and produces dynamic hyperinflation, thus leading to increased work in breathing and symptoms of breathlessness. Lung volume reduction surgery seems to affect those changes, probably through a combination of improvement of lung recoil, changes in lung size and its effects on respiratory muscles. Lung volume reduction surgery involves resection of emphysematous lung with the aim of reducing lung volume. In recent years non-surgical procedures, in the form of endobronchial valve insertion, have become more widely used. The Valve for Emphysema Palliation Trial (VENT) compared endobronchial valve placement with best medical therapy (Sciurba et al. 2010). The endobronchial valves were placed unilaterally in the lobes that had the worst emphysema. Results showed that at 6 months there was significant increase of FEV_1 by 60 ml and the 6 minutes walk by 19.1 meters (5.8%) in the endobrocnhial valve group compared with the medical treatment group. The other important finding of the VENT study was that patients with intra-lobar heterogeneous emphysema of more than 15% and the presence of complete fissures had the best improvements in FEV_1 and the 6 minute walk. The IMPACT study showed that patients with homogenous emphysema and who had no collateral ventilation in the targeted lobes can also benefit from endobronchial valve treatment (Valipour et al. 2016). The benefits observed were related to improvements in the FEV_1, 6 minutes walk and quality of life. Similarly, the STELVIO study showed significant improvement in patients with emphysema who had endobronchial valve insertion compared with the control group at 6 months in mean FEV_1 measurements by 178% and mean 6 minutes walk distance by 23.3% (Hartman et al. 2018, Klooster, Hartman, et al. 2017). In the LIBERATE study, endobronchial valves were evaluated in patients with heterogenous emphysema and little or no collateral ventilation in the target lobe, showing improvement in lung function, exercise tolerance and St George's Respiratory Questionnaire scores (Criner et al. 2018). In the endobronchial valve group the improvements in FEV_1 were 0.106 L ($p < 0.001$), 6 minutes walk of 39.31 meters ($p = 0.002$) and for St George's Respiratory Questionnaire Score reduction by 7.05 points ($p = 0.004$). Pneumothorax was observed in 26% of cases.

Endoscopic lung volume reduction can be performed using a flexible bronchoscope. This form of treatment can be used for patients with severe COPD who have been carefully assessed. The currently accepted criteria for endoscopic lung volume reduction include FEV_1 ranging from 15% to 50% of predicted and residual volume of more than 175% of predicted (Herth et al. 2017). Patients should be advised to stop smoking, their medication should be maximized and they should have been through a pulmonary rehabilitation process. In addition, the patients should be stable prior to procedure and should be able to undergo general anesthesia or awake sedation. Radiological imaging should exclude other pathologies and provide evidence of the presence of complete fissures. In some cases, imaging may not be able to definitively confirm the absence of collateral ventilation in the lobes targeted for endobronchial valve insertion, even using more advanced imaging technology. For this reason the most accepted method for precisely assessing collateral ventilation status is the Chartis Diagnostic System (Pulmonx) (Slebos et al. 2017). The procedure of endoscopic valve insertion and the Chartis measurements are recommended to be performed under general anesthesia as this allows for better airway management. There are recommended settings of ventilation, such as low ventilation frequency and long expiratory settings as, these are less likely to affect the Chartis measurements (Slebos et al. 2017). During the Chartis procedure, patients require adequate levels of sedation whilst still being able to produce tidal breathing for negative collateral ventilation to be detected. However, because the patients have advanced COPD, during the procedure they need to be monitored for respiratory failure and carbon dioxide retention. Therefore, sedation used needs to be easily reversible; most commonly, agents used are short acting benzodiazepines and opiates. Similarly, good secretion management is of importance. The use of positive pressure ventilation is recommended for both the Chartis measurements and the placement of the valves. Although the procedure can be performed under awake sedation there are clear advantages of general anesthesia and positive pressure ventilation (Slebos et al. 2017, Shah et al. 2017). The patient is more comfortable; coughing and the management of secretions may be easier. In fact, if Chartis assessment is inconclusive under awake sedation, measurements may be improved when performed under general anaesthesia, especially in patients who have fissure completeness above 80%. In addition, it is recommended that Chartis measurements and the placement of valves is undertaken at the same time, thus reducing the risks of COPD exacerbation due to repeat bronchoscopies if procedures were performed separately.

The decision where to place the endobronchial valve is determined by imaging that locates the distribution of disease and characterizes fissures, as well as findings of the Chartis measurements. Imaging characteristics of the targeted lobes should include assessment for the presence of fissures, absence of collateral ventilation, presence of emphysema and low perfusion on perfusion scintigraphy (Slebos and Shah 2016, Koegelenberg et al. 2015, Herth et al. 2016). Valve placement also needs to take into consideration careful assessment of the bronchial anatomy. This should consider the size of the bronchi as well as their proximity, since this determines the order of the valve placement. It is normal practice to first place valves in the more distal bronchi to avoid valve overlap, which may prevent placement of subsequent valves into the more distal segments. The depth marker on the endobronchial delivery catheter allows assessment of the distance of valve protrusion post placement.

The most common complications of insertion of endobronchial valve include pneumothorax, infection and misplacement of the valve (Herth et al. 2017, Slebos et al. 2017). These complications require rapid intervention, such as treatment of infection; this would usually involve nebulised bronchodilators, systemic corticosteroids and antibiotics. Pneumothorax has been reported to occur in around 20 to 30% of cases

(Klooster et al. 2015, Klooster, Slebos, et al. 2017). The majority, around 80% of cases of pneumothorax, occur in the first 2 days post procedure, with one in ten occurring after 6 days and around 10% between day 3 and 5 post procedure (Skowasch et al. 2016). The management of pneumothorax should follow international guidelines and involve rapid chest drain insertion to avoid tension pneumothorax (MacDuff, Arnold, and Harvey 2010). There are currently two endobronchial valve systems: Zephyr that has been more widely used and Spiration endobronchial valve. There are other options such as self-acting coils, use of biodegradeable sclerosant or thermal vapour.

Endobronchial Ultrasound

Mediastinoscopy is the gold standard for mediastinal lymph node staging in the context of lung cancer. Imaging, such as computed tomography (CT), Positron Emission Tomography (PET) or Magnetic Resonance Imaging (MRI) in some cases, provide non-invasive methods for mediastinal lymph node staging (Whitson et al. 2013, Rintoul et al. 2009). Other options for staging mediastinal lymph nodes include Endobronchial Ultrasound (EBUS), Endoscopic Ultrasound (EUS) or blind Trans-Bronchial Fine Needle Aspiration (TBFNA) sampling. CT and PET can identify mediastinal lymph node involvement in NSCLC with sensitivity of 60% to 85%, specificity of 84% to 94% and accuracy of 78% to 96% (Groth and Andrade 2008). Cervical mediastinoscopy has sensitivity of 86% to 93% and diagnostic accuracy of 93% to 96% (Annema et al. 2010, Yasufuku et al. 2011). It has been reported to have morbidity of 0.6% to 1.1% (Hammoud et al. 1999). EBUS is a less invasive procedure compared with cervical mediastinoscopy and can be performed under awake sedation as well as under general anaesthesia.

Accurate staging of lung cancer is important for prognostic and therapeutic reasons. EBUS was introduced in the early 1990's. The early technology introduced a radial probe, which allowed for visualization of the airway wall with close proximity to the exterior of the airways (Herth,

Becker, and Ernst 2003). With improvement, it allowed for the use of a radial probe with a flexible catheter and a balloon to perform biopsies, including transbronchial needle aspiration but not real time procedures. Convex probe development resulted in the ability to perform real time visualization of the lymph nodes with real time ability to biopsy lymph nodes. EBUS, using a convex probe allows for lymph node staging and biopsy, diagnosis of mediastinal tumours and diagnosis of lymph nodes of unknown aetiology, for example in the context of undiagnosed TB or sarcoid, or biopsy of a pulmonary neoplasm (Gompelmann, Eberhardt, and Herth 2012, Herth and Eberhardt 2007). The EBUS convex probe is a 7.5 MHz transducer, placed at the tip of the scope; it is a linear, curved array scanning parallel to the scope insertion. The images are produced by directly contacting the probe with the bronchial wall, or they can be enhanced by attaching a balloon to the end of the scope. The scope also allows for visualization of the bronchial tree with conventional flexible bronchoscopy imaging. EBUS can also use Doppler mode to identify blood vessels. Radial probe EBUS can be used to assess the airway wall and its layers and to localize lymph nodes close to the trachea and bronchi, thus allowing subsequent lymph node biopsies, though not under real time ultrasound guidance, to localize lung lesions and subsequently guide placement of a guide sheath for biopsy. EBUS allows for a 22-gauge needle to be inserted through the working channel allowing for real time ultrasound guided transbronchial needle aspiration.

EBUS can be performed under general anaesthesia with an 8.5 mm or larger endotracheal tube as EBUS is slightly larger than a conventional fiberoptic bronchoscope. The endotracheal tube should be placed just below the glottis to allow for good apposition against the tracheal wall to provide good quality of images. This is of particular importance when sampling station 2 lymph nodes. The advantages of general anaesthesia include better control of oxygenation, improved sampling of smaller lymph nodes - less than 10 mm in diameter - by using intermittent apnoea, thus reducing patients' movement. The main disadvantages include the possible side effects of the anaesthetic agents, including hypotension and nausea, trauma from intubation and a longer recovery time. There was no difference in outcomes of EBUS performed under general anaesthesia compared with EBUS performed under conscious sedation, with reported sensitivity of 94.8% and 94% and 94% accuracy of EBUS performed under GA and conscious sedation respectively (Gompelmann, Eberhardt, and Herth 2012, Herth and Eberhardt 2007). Numerous studies have reported EBUS and EUS as relatively safe procedures with reported serious complications ranging between 0.05% to 1.43% (von Bartheld, van Breda, and Annema 2014). The most commonly reported complications, which are relatively minor, include cough, low oxygen levels that improve post procedure and, occasionally, high temperature which is self-limiting or may require antibiotic therapy.

EBUS can access American Thoracic Society (ATS) stations 2, 3, 4, 7, 10, 11; mediastinoscopy can sample stations 1, 2, 3, 4, 7 and EUS stations 2L, 4L, 7, 8, 9 (Groth and Andrade 2008). Using a fiberoptic bronchoscope mediastinal lymph nodes can be sampled but this is performed without direct visualization and was, not surprisingly, reported to have a wide diagnostic yield ranging between 40 to 75% (Groth and Andrade 2008). This inconsistency in diagnostic yield is the main disadvantage of the TBFNA. In a randomized controlled study EBUS diagnostic yield was 80%, which was statistically significant higher compared with that of TBFNA of 71% ($p < 0.005$) (Herth, Becker, and Ernst 2004). The use of the linear probe allows for real time procedure, with EBUS reported sensitivity of 89% to 99% and a diagnostic yield of 85% to 99% (Herth, Eberhardt, et al. 2006, Herth, Ernst, et al. 2006). Dong et al. performed a meta-analysis, which pooled results from 1066 patients who had both EBUS and surgical analysis of the lymph nodes, revealing sensitivity of 0.90 (CI 0.84 to 0.96) (Dong et al. 2013). The findings were not greatly dissimilar to the earlier meta-analysis (Gu et al. 2009). Yasufuku et al, in a randomized controlled study which analyzed EBUS and mediastinoscopy for assessment of nodal staging, showed that both procedures had similar diagnostic accuracy of 93%, with no difference in sensitivity and negative predictive values (Yasufuku et al. 2011). In contrast, Um et al. reported, in a prospective study of 127 patients who had both EBUS and mediastinoscopy, a significantly higher 93% accuracy for EBUS compared with that of 89% for mediastinoscopy (Um et al. 2015). However, Annema et al. in a randomized controlled study, compared surgical staging with that performed with EBUS and EUS, showing that surgical sensitivity for detection of cancer was 79% and was similar to that of 85% for combined EBUS and EUS (Annema et al. 2010). The important finding of this study was that mediastinoscopy increased sensitivity by 9% if performed in cases where EBUS/EUS node sampling showed no evidence of cancer. In another study, Liberman et al. prospectively assessed 166 patients already diagnosed or investigated for suspected lung cancer who underwent EBU/EUS and surgical mediastinal staging in the same setting and reported that EBUS had diagnostic accuracy of 91%, EUS of 88% and combined EBUS/EUS of 97% (Liberman et al. 2014). Therefore, based on currently available research EBUS has similar or slightly higher diagnostic yield when compared with mediastinoscopy. Moreover, combining EBUS with EUS may increase the diagnostic yield.

When performing EBUS, the planning of the procedure should be undertaken based on the most recent imaging, including CT and PET. It is good practice not only to review the images with respect to the lymph node characteristics and FDG uptake but also to compare radiological measurements of the lymph nodes with those of EBUS. Once the appropriate lymph nodes are visualized, a biopsy can be performed under real time. 10 to 15 needle passes are recommended and each lymph node should be sampled 1 to 3 times depending on the size of sample obtained (Gompelmann, Eberhardt, and Herth 2012). Many centers perform on site cytology analysis, which allows for decision whether the samples obtained are adequate to provide diagnosis; the decision can then be made whether additional sampling is required. Current practice is that samples should be sufficient for mutation testing, as systemic therapy requires analysis for EGFR, ALK and PD-L1. There are important issues related to the cytological analysis of the collected samples. The presence of lymphocytes can assist confirmation that the lymph node was sampled and is predictive of adequate sampling; the absence of lymphocytes has a negative predictive value for adequacy of sampling. There are potential issues of bronchial contamination that may result in false positive results. Sampling of the lymph nodes should be performed from more proximal to more distal e.g., N3 nodes followed by N2 nodes followed by N1 nodes as, otherwise, there is potential for contamination and upstaging of disease. EBUS can also be used for the diagnosis of sarcoidosis, TB or metastatic cancer from other sites. In cases of suspected TB, samples are required to be sent for histology and cytology, as well as microbiology and mycobacterial cultures. In some cases of chronic sarcoidosis where the nodes are fibrotic, a mediastinoscopy may be required for diagnosis. The role of EBUS in diagnosing lymphoma is not clear as diagnostic yield is variable; therefore, surgical biopsy may be more appropriate.

The learning curve for EBUS is variable even for the experienced bronchoscopists (Kemp et al. 2010). There is evidence that diagnostic yield of 90% can be achieved with around 50 procedures (Bellinger et al. 2014). Overall the learning curve depends on which node stations are sampled. For example, identification and sampling of stations significant in size, 7 subcarinal or para-tracheal 4R or 4L, would be much easier to master than small hilar nodes. In experienced hands even less than 5 mm nodes can be sampled. The American College of Chest Physicians (ACCP) recommends at least 50 procedures to establish proficiency in EBUS (Ernst, Silvestri, and Johnstone 2003). The ATS and European Respiratory Society (ERS) recommend at least 40 procedures under supervision (Bolliger et al. 2002). Others have observed that the learning curve was 10 procedures (Groth et al. 2008). The learning curve can be improved by the use of simulation training (Stather et al. 2012).

Virtual Bronchoscopic Navigation

Virtual bronchoscopic navigation, also called navigational bronchoscopy, involves the use of flexible bronchoscopy guided by virtual bronchoscopy to reach peripheral lung lesions (Asano, Eberhardt, and Herth 2014, Silvestri et al. 2012). Navigational bronchoscopy, when used with an ultra thin computed tomography, has been reported to have a diagnostic yield of between 65.4% to 81.6% (Asano, Eberhardt, and Herth

2014). When using an EBUS guided sheath, the diagnostic yield from the sampling of peripheral lesions has been reported at between 63.3% and 84.4%. The use of virtual bronchoscopy compared to the EBUS guided sheath improved the diagnostic yield. The navigational bronchoscopy has its advantages as, for an experienced bronchoscopist, there is very short learning curve which may not require additional training. The procedure is shorter compared to the EBUS guided sheath therefore associated with improved patient comfort with low complication rate, around 1% (Asano, Eberhardt, and Herth 2014). The main disadvantages are related to relatively high costs of the equipment which is the main limiting factor (Asano, Eberhardt, and Herth 2014, Silvestri et al. 2012).

Conclusion

In conclusion, due to technological improvements there have been interesting developments in the field of bronchoscopy. The use of new technologies has been applied in investigational procedures such as mediastinal nodes sampling using EBUS, thus reducing the need for mediastinoscopy. Moreover, navigational bronchoscopy may become more widely used for sampling of peripheral lung lesions. This new technique can be undertaken and easily learned by experienced bronchoscopists. Similarly, insertion of endobronchial valves for patients with emphysema, or those with persistent air leak, are performed using flexible bronchoscopy. There is no doubt that, together with technological advances, new bronchoscopic techniques will be developed, widening the application of diagnostic and therapeutic bronchoscopic options.

References

Akopov, A. L., Rusanov, A. A. Papayan, G. V. Kazakov, N. V. Gerasin, A. V. and Urtenova, M. A. 2017. "Endobronchial photodynamic therapy under fluorescence control: Photodynamic theranostics." *Photodiagnosis Photodyn Ther* no. 19:73-77. doi: 10.1016/j. pdpdt.2017.05.001.

Allison, R. R., and Moghissi, K. 2013. "Oncologic photodynamic therapy: clinical strategies that modulate mechanisms of action." *Photodiagnosis Photodyn Ther* no. 10 (4):331-41. doi: 10.1016/ j.pdpdt.2013.03.011.

Annema, J. T., van Meerbeeck, J. P., Rintoul, R. C., Dooms, C., Deschepper, E., Dekkers, O. M., De Leyn, P., Braun, J., Carroll, N. R. Praet, M., dc Ryck, F., Vansteenkiste, J., Vermassen, F,. Versteegh, M. I., Veselic, M., Nicholson, A. G., Rabe, K. F., and Tournoy, K. G. 2010. "Mediastinoscopy vs endosonography for mediastinal nodal staging of lung cancer: a randomized trial." *JAMA* no. 304 (20):2245-52. doi: 10.1001/jama.2010.1705.

Annigeri, R. V., and Patil, R. S. 2017. "A Retrospective Analysis on Anesthetic Management during Rigid Bronchoscopy in Children with Foreign Body Aspiration: Propofol and Sevoflurane with Controlled Ventilation." *Anesth Essays Res* no. 11 (4):871-874. doi: 10.4103/aer. AER_154_17.

Asano, F., Eberhardt, R., and Herth, F. J. 2014. "Virtual bronchoscopic navigation for peripheral pulmonary lesions." *Respiration* no. 88 (5):430-40. doi: 10.1159/000367900.

Batra, H., and Yarmus, L. 2018. "Indications and complications of rigid bronchoscopy." *Expert Rev Respir Med* no. 12 (6):509-520. doi: 10.1080/17476348.2018.1473037.

Bellinger, C. R., Chatterjee, A. B., Adair, N., Houle, T., Khan, I. and Haponik, E. 2014. "Training in and experience with endobronchial ultrasound." *Respiration* no. 88 (6):478-83. doi: 10.1159/000368366.

Blum, M. G., Powers, T. W. and Sundaresan, S. 2004. "Bronchoscopy simulator effectively prepares junior residents to competently perform basic clinical bronchoscopy." *Ann Thorac Surg* no. 78 (1):287-91; discussion 287-91. doi: 10.1016/j.athoracsur.2003.11.058.

Bolliger, C. T., Mathur, P. N., Beamis, J. F., Becker, H. D., Cavaliere, S., Colt, H., Diaz-Jimenez, J. P., Dumon, J. F., Edell, E., Kovitz, K. L., Macha, H. N., Mehta, A. C., Marel, M., Noppen, M., Strausz, J., and

Sutedja, T. G. 2002. "ERS/ATS statement on interventional pulmonology. European Respiratory Society/American Thoracic Society." *Eur Respir J* no. 19 (2):356-73.

Criner, G. J., Sue, R. Wright, S. Dransfield, M. Rivas-Perez, H. Wiese, T. Sciurba, F. C. Shah, P. L. Wahidi, M. M. de Oliveira, H. G. Morrissey, B. Cardoso, P. F. G. Hays, S. Majid, A. Pastis, Jr., N. Kopas, L. Vollenweider, M. McFadden, P. M. Machuzak, M. Hsia, D. W. Sung, A., Jarad, N., Kornaszewska, M., Hazelrigg, S., Krishna, G,. Armstrong, B., Shargill, N. S., and Slebos, D. J. 2018. "A Multicenter RCT of Zephyr(R) Endobronchial Valve Treatment in Heterogeneous Emphysema (LIBERATE)." *Am J Respir Crit Care Med*. doi: 10.1164/rccm.201803-0590OC.

Davoudi, M., and H. G. Colt. 2009. "Bronchoscopy simulation: a brief review." *Adv Health Sci Educ Theory Pract* no. 14 (2):287-96. doi: 10.1007/s10459-007-9095-x.

Dong, X., X. Qiu, Q. Liu, and J. Jia. 2013. "Endobronchial ultrasound-guided transbronchial needle aspiration in the mediastinal staging of non-small cell lung cancer: a meta-analysis." *Ann Thorac Surg* no. 96 (4):1502-7. doi: 10.1016/j.athoracsur.2013.05.016.

Du Rand, I. A., Barber, P. V., Goldring, J., Lewis, R. A., Mandal, S., Munavvar, M., Rintoul, R. C., Shah, P. L., Singh, S., Slade, M. G., and Woolley, A. 2011. "British Thoracic Society guideline for advanced diagnostic and therapeutic flexible bronchoscopy in adults." *Thorax* no. 66 Suppl 3:iii1-21. doi: 10.1136/thoraxjnl-2011-200713.

Du Rand, I. A., Blaikley, J. Booton, R. Chaudhuri, N. Gupta, V. Khalid, S. Mandal, S. Martin, J. Mills, J. Navani, N. Rahman, N. M. Wrightson, J. M. and Munavvar, M. 2013. "British Thoracic Society guideline for diagnostic flexible bronchoscopy in adults: accredited by NICE." *Thorax* no. 68 Suppl 1:i1-i44. doi: 10.1136/thoraxjnl-2013-203618.

Ernst, A., Silvestri, G. A., and Johnstone, D. 2003. "Interventional pulmonary procedures: Guidelines from the American College of Chest Physicians." *Chest* no. 123 (5):1693-717.

Gompelmann, D., Eberhardt, R., and Herth, F. J. 2012. "Endobronchial ultrasound." *Endosc Ultrasound* no. 1 (2):69-74. doi: 10.7178/eus.02.003.

Groth, S. S., and Andrade, R. S. 2008. "Endobronchial ultrasound-guided transbronchial needle aspiration for mediastinal lymph node staging in non-small cell lung cancer." *Semin Thorac Cardiovasc Surg* no. 20 (4):274-8. doi: 10.1053/j.semtcvs.2008.11.004.

Groth, S. S., Whitson, B. A., D'Cunha, J., Maddaus, M. A., Alsharif, M., and Andrade, R. S. 2008. "Endobronchial ultrasound-guided fine-needle aspiration of mediastinal lymph nodes: a single institution's early learning curve." *Ann Thorac Surg* no. 86 (4):1104-9; discussion 1109-10. doi: 10.1016/j.athoracsur.2008.06.042.

Gu, P., Y. Z. Zhao, L. Y. Jiang, W. Zhang, Y. Xin, and B. H. Han. 2009. "Endobronchial ultrasound-guided transbronchial needle aspiration for staging of lung cancer: a systematic review and meta-analysis." *Eur J Cancer* no. 45 (8):1389-96. doi: 10.1016/j.ejca.2008.11.043.

Hammoud, Z. T., Anderson, R. C., Meyers, B. F., Guthrie, T. J., Roper, C. L., Cooper, J. D., and Patterson, G. A. 1999. "The current role of mediastinoscopy in the evaluation of thoracic disease." *J Thorac Cardiovasc Surg* no. 118 (5):894-9.

Haponik, E. F., Russell, G. B., Beamis, Jr., J. F., Britt, E. J., Kvale, P., Mathur, P., and Mehta, A. 2000. "Bronchoscopy training: current fellows' experiences and some concerns for the future." *Chest* no. 118 (3):625-30.

Hartman, J. E., Klooster, K., Groen, H., Ten Hacken, N. H. T., and Slebos, D. J. 2018. "Cost-effectiveness of endobronchial valve treatment in patients with severe emphysema compared to standard medical care." *Respirology*. doi: 10.1111/resp.13295.

Herth, F., Becker, H. D., and Ernst, A. 2004. "Conventional vs endobronchial ultrasound-guided transbronchial needle aspiration: a randomized trial." *Chest* no. 125 (1):322-5.

Herth, F. J., Becker, H. D., and Ernst, A., 2003. "Ultrasound-guided transbronchial needle aspiration: an experience in 242 patients." *Chest* no. 123 (2):604-7.

Herth, F. J., and Eberhardt, R., 2007. "Actual role of endobronchial ultrasound (EBUS)." *Eur Radiol* no. 17 (7):1806-12. doi: 10.1007/s00330-006-0497-6.

Herth, F. J., Eberhardt, R., Vilmann, P., Krasnik, M., and Ernst, A., 2006. "Real-time endobronchial ultrasound guided transbronchial needle aspiration for sampling mediastinal lymph nodes." *Thorax* no. 61 (9):795-8. doi: 10.1136/thx.2005.047829.

Herth, F. J., Ernst, A., Eberhardt, R., Vilmann, P., Dienemann, H., and Krasnik, M., 2006. "Endobronchial ultrasound-guided transbronchial needle aspiration of lymph nodes in the radiologically normal mediastinum." *Eur Respir J* no. 28 (5):910-4. doi: 10.1183/09031936.06.00124905.

Herth, F. J. F., D. J. Slebos, G. J. Criner, and P. L. Shah. 2017. "Endoscopic Lung Volume Reduction: An Expert Panel Recommendation - Update 2017." *Respiration* no. 94 (4):380-388. doi: 10.1159/000479379.

Herth, F. J., Slebos, D. J., Rabe, K. F., and Shah, P. L. 2016. "Endoscopic Lung Volume Reduction: An Expert Panel Recommendation." *Respiration* no. 91 (3):241-50. doi: 10.1159/000444090.

Ikeda, N., Usuda, J., Kato, H., Ishizumi, T., Ichinose, S., Otani, K., Honda, H., Furukawa, K., Okunaka, T., and Tsutsui, H. 2011. "New aspects of photodynamic therapy for central type early stage lung cancer." *Lasers Surg Med* no. 43 (7):749-54. doi: 10.1002/lsm.21091.

Kemp, S. V., El Batrawy, S. H., Harrison, R. N., Skwarski, K., Munavvar, M., Rosell, A., Cusworth, K., and Shah, P. L. 2010. "Learning curves for endobronchial ultrasound using cusum analysis." *Thorax* no. 65 (6):534-8. doi: 10.1136/thx.2009.127274.

Klooster, K., Hartman, J. E., Ten Hacken, N. H., and Slebos, D. J. 2017. "One-Year Follow-Up after Endobronchial Valve Treatment in Patients with Emphysema without Collateral Ventilation Treated in the STELVIO Trial." *Respiration* no. 93 (2):112-121. doi: 10.1159/000453529.

Klooster, K., Slebos, D. J., Zoumot, Z., Davey, C., Shah, P. L., and Hopkinson, N. S. 2017. "Endobronchial valves for emphysema: an individual patient-level reanalysis of randomised controlled trials." *BMJ Open Respir Res* no. 4 (1):e000214. doi: 10.1136/bmjresp-2017-000214.

Klooster, K., ten Hacken, N. H., Hartman, J. E., Kerstjens, H. A., van Rikxoort, E. M., and Slebos, D. J. 2015. "Endobronchial Valves for Emphysema without Interlobar Collateral Ventilation." *N Engl J Med* no. 373 (24):2325-35. doi: 10.1056/NEJMoa1507807.

Koegelenberg, C. F., Theron, J., Dheda, K., Bruwer, J. W., Allwood, B. W., Vorster, M. J., von Groote-Bidlingmaier, F., Slebos, D. J., Shah, P. L., and Herth, F. J. 2015. "Recommendations for the use of endoscopic lung volume reduction in South Africa: Role in the treatment of emphysema." *S Afr Med J* no. 105 (10):810-5. doi: 10.7196/SAMJ new.8147.

Kvale, P. A., and Mehta, A. C. 2001. "Training bronchoscopists for the new era." *Clin Chest Med* no. 22 (2):365-72, ix.

Liberman, M., J. Sampalis, A. Duranceau, V. Thiffault, R. Hadjeres, and P. Ferraro. 2014. "Endosonographic mediastinal lymph node staging of lung cancer." *Chest* no. 146 (2):389-397. doi: 10.1378/chest.13-2349.

MacDuff, A., Arnold, A., and Harvey, J., 2010. "Management of spontaneous pneumothorax: British Thoracic Society Pleural Disease Guideline 2010." *Thorax* no. 65 Suppl 2:ii18-31. doi: 10.1136/thx. 2010.136986.

Mehta, A. C., Hood, K. L., Schwarz, Y., and Solomon, S. B. 2018. "The Evolutional History of Electromagnetic Navigation Bronchoscopy: State of the Art." *Chest*. doi: 10.1016/j.chest.2018.04.029.

Moghissi, K., and Dixon, K. 2003. "Is bronchoscopic photodynamic therapy a therapeutic option in lung cancer?" *Eur Respir J* no. 22 (3):535-41.

Moghissi, K., and Dixon, K. 2008. "Update on the current indications, practice and results of photodynamic therapy (PDT) in early central lung cancer (ECLC)." *Photodiagnosis Photodyn Ther* no. 5 (1):10-8. doi: 10.1016/j.pdpdt.2007.11.001.

Moghissi, K., and Dixon, K. 2017. "Photodynamic therapy (PDT) for adenoid cystic carcinoma of the tracheo-bronchial tree: Report of 4 cases." *Photodiagnosis Photodyn Ther* no. 18:95-97. doi: 10.1016/j.pdpdt.2017.02.002.

Moghissi, K., Dixon, K., Stringer, M., Freeman, T., Thorpe, A., and Brown, S. 1999. "The place of bronchoscopic photodynamic therapy in advanced unresectable lung cancer: experience of 100 cases." *Eur J Cardiothorac Surg* no. 15 (1):1-6.

Moghissi, K., Dixon, K., Thorpe, J. A., Stringer, M., and Oxtoby, C. 2007. "Photodynamic therapy (PDT) in early central lung cancer: a treatment option for patients ineligible for surgical resection." *Thorax* no. 62 (5):391-5. doi: 10.1136/thx.2006.061143.

Okunaka, T., and Kato, H. 2002. "[Photodynamic therapy for lung cancer: state of the art and expanded indications]." *Nihon Geka Gakkai Zasshi* no. 103 (2):258-62.

Rayl, J. E., Pittman, J. M., and Shuster, J. J. 1988. "Preclinical training in bronchoscopic diagnosis of cancer." *Chest* no. 93 (4):824-7.

Rintoul, R. C., Tournoy, K. G., El Daly, H., Carroll, N. R., Buttery, R. C., van Kralingen, K., van Meerbeeck, J. P., Rabe, K. F., and Annema J. T. 2009. "EBUS-TBNA for the clarification of PET positive intra-thoracic lymph nodes-an international multi-centre experience." *J Thorac Oncol* no. 4 (1):44-8. doi: 10.1097/JTO.0b013e3181914357.

Ross, P., Jr., Grecula, J., Bekaii-Saab, T., Villalona-Calero, M., Otterson, G., and Magro C. 2006. "Incorporation of photodynamic therapy as an induction modality in non-small cell lung cancer." *Lasers Surg Med* no. 38 (10):881-9. doi: 10.1002/lsm.20444.

Sciurba, F. C., Ernst, A., Herth, F. J., Strange, C., Criner, G. J., Marquette, C. H., Kovitz, K. L., Chiacchierini, R. P., Goldin, J., and McLennan, G. 2010. "A randomized study of endobronchial valves for advanced emphysema." *N Engl J Med* no. 363 (13):1233-44. doi: 10.1056/NEJMoa0900928.

Shah, P. L., Herth, F. J., van Geffen, W. H., Deslee, G., and Slebos, D. J. 2017. "Lung volume reduction for emphysema." *Lancet Respir Med* no. 5 (2):147-156. doi: 10.1016/s2213-2600(16)30221-1.

Silvestri, G. A. 2008. "The evolution of bronchoscopy training." *Respiration* no. 76 (1):19-20. doi: 10.1159/000127579.

Silvestri, G. A., Feller-Kopman, D., Chen, A., Wahidi, M., Yasufuku, K., and Ernst, A. 2012. "Latest advances in advanced diagnostic and therapeutic pulmonary procedures." *Chest* no. 142 (6):1636-44. doi: 10.1378/chest.12-2326.

Skowasch, D., Fertl, A., Schwick, B., Schafer, H., Hellmann, A., and Herth, F. J. 2016. "A Long-Term Follow-Up Investigation of Endobronchial Valves in Emphysema (the LIVE Study): Study Protocol and Six-Month Interim Analysis Results of a Prospective Five-Year Observational Study." *Respiration* no. 92 (2):118-26. doi: 10.1159/000448119.

Slebos, D. J., and Shah, P. L. 2016. "Go with the Flow: The Importance of the Assessment of Collateral Ventilation in Endobronchial Valve Treatment." *Respiration* no. 91 (4):269-70. doi: 10.1159/000444330.

Slebos, D. J., Shah, P. L., Herth, F. J., and Valipour, A.2017. "Endobronchial Valves for Endoscopic Lung Volume Reduction: Best Practice Recommendations from Expert Panel on Endoscopic Lung Volume Reduction." *Respiration* no. 93 (2):138-150. doi: 10.1159/000453588.

Stather, D. R., MacEachern, P., Chee, A., Dumoulin, E., and Tremblay, A. 2012. "Evaluation of clinical endobronchial ultrasound skills following clinical versus simulation training." *Respirology* no. 17 (2):291-9. doi: 10.1111/j.1440-1843.2011.02068.x.

Torrington, K. G. 2000. "Bronchoscopy training and competency: how many are enough?" *Chest* no. 118 (3):572-3.

Um, S. W., Kim, H. K., Jung, S. H., Han, J., Lee, K. J., Park, H. Y., Choi, Y. S., Shim, Y. M., Ahn, M. J., Park, K., Ahn, Y. C., Choi, J. Y., Lee, K. S., Suh, G. Y., Chung, M. P., Kwon, O. J., Kim, J., and Kim, H. 2015. "Endobronchial ultrasound versus mediastinoscopy for mediastinal nodal staging of non-small-cell lung cancer." *J Thorac Oncol* no. 10 (2):331-7. doi: 10.1097/jto.0000000000000388.

Valipour, A., Slebos, D. J., Herth, F., Darwiche, K. Wagner, M., Ficker, J. H., Petermann, C., Hubner, R. H., Stanzel, F., and Eberhardt, R. 2016. "Endobronchial Valve Therapy in Patients with Homogeneous

Emphysema. Results from the IMPACT Study." *Am J Respir Crit Care Med* no. 194 (9):1073-1082. doi: 10.1164/rccm.201607-1383OC.

von Bartheld, M. B., van Breda, A., and Annema, J. T. 2014. "Complication rate of endosonography (endobronchial and endoscopic ultrasound): a systematic review." *Respiration* no. 87 (4):343-51. doi: 10.1159/000357066.

Wahidi, M. M., Jain, P., Jantz, M., Lee, P., Mackensen, G. B., Barbour, S. Y., Lamb, C., and Silvestri, G. A. 2011. "American College of Chest Physicians consensus statement on the use of topical anesthesia, analgesia, and sedation during flexible bronchoscopy in adult patients." *Chest* no. 140 (5):1342-50. doi: 10.1378/chest.10-3361.

Whitson, B. A., Groth, S. S., Odell, D. D., Briones, E. P., Maddaus, M. A., D'Cunha, J., and Andrade, R. S. 2013. "True negative predictive value of endobronchial ultrasound in lung cancer: are we being conservative enough?" *Ann Thorac Surg* no. 95 (5):1689-94. doi: 10.1016/j.athoracsur.2012.09.057.

Yasufuku, K., Pierre, A., Darling, G., de Perrot, M., Waddell, T., Johnston, M., da Cunha Santos, G., Geddie, W., Boerner, S., Le, L. W., and Keshavjee, S. 2011. "A prospective controlled trial of endobronchial ultrasound-guided transbronchial needle aspiration compared with mediastinoscopy for mediatinal lymph node staging of lung cancer." *J Thorac Cardiovasc Surg* no. 142 (6):1393-400 e1. doi: 10.1016/j.jtcvs.2011.08.037.

In: Handbook of Surgical Procedures
Editor: Heather Gilbert
ISBN: 978-1-53614-580-9

Chapter 4

Postoperative Pancreatic Fistula Following Distal Pancreatectomy

Jennifer L. Olson, MD and Richard J. Bold*, MD
Division of Surgical Oncology,
UC Davis Comprehensive Cancer Center, Sacramento, CA, US

1. Introduction

Post-operative pancreatic fistula (POPF) is one of the most dreaded complications in any pancreatic operation given its associated morbidity and mortality. The amylase-rich fluid can cause inflammation, become infected, or cause serious bleeding from neighboring vasculature. POPF are at least as common after distal pancreatectomy than traditional pancreaticoduodenectomy, occurring in approximately 14-30% of all operations [1-3]. Unlike pancreaticoduodenectomy, there is no pancreatic ductal anastomosis at risk for leakage and disruption; it has been hypothesized that the intact sphincter of Oddi as well as the normal parenchymal texture accounts for the relatively high incidence of POPF

* Correspondence Author Email: rjbold@ucdavis.edu.

including the splanchnic vessels leading to major hemorrhage. When bacteria are introduced into the fluid collection, an intraabdominal abscess can lead to sepsis. In a retrospective analysis of 908 patients who underwent pancreatic resection, culture of the pancreatic fistula effluent revealed bacteria in 2/3 of the patients [9]. Organisms are almost always gram-negative rods or anaerobes which likely represent enteric bacterial translocation or seeding at the time of the operation [10]. Mortality attributed to complicated POPF are as high as 5% [9].

Oncologic outcomes are also influenced. Prolonged hospitalization and convalescence delay initiation of chemotherapy. Whether due to the delay or absence of adjuvant systemic therapy, or the impact of the complication on overall health status, recurrence-free survival for pancreatic adenocarcinoma is decreased after POPF [11].

4. Patient Factors

Many patient factors have been shown to predispose patients to POPF. Some are disputed such as increased BMI and malignancy [12-14]. Malignancy is reported to both increase and decrease the rate of POPF. It can alter the gland by enlarging the duct after an obstructive process facilitating identification for directed ligation. The pancreatic gland following neoadjuvant radiation is more fibrotic/firm and may be associated with a lower POPF. Pancreatic texture is widely accepted as a risk factor with a firm pancreas conferring a lower risk compared to a soft gland texture [3, 4]. Texture is a subjective assessment of soft and firm that cannot be determined prior to the operation and attempts to define texture radiographically have not been successful [15]. Poor nutritional status by different measures may increase POPF risk although it doesn't stand up to multivariable analysis and the difference of albumin between groups is subclinical [12, 16]. Knowledge of patient factors influencing POPF does not change patient selection but may influence preoperative counseling and post-operative decision making.

5. Surgical Techniques

5.1. Approach

Distal pancreatectomy can be performed open, laparoscopically, or robotically. The laparoscopic approach is popular given the advantages in hospitalization and recovery time for minimally invasive surgery. Given the absence of required anastomoses to create, the technical feasibility is within the scope for most pancreatic surgeons. Several studies have compared outcomes including POPF and have shown that the laparoscopic and robotic approach are safe. [15, 17-20].

5.2. Division

Division of the pancreas can be performed by scalpel, stapler, or energy device in an open surgery and stapler or energy device in a minimally invasive approach. There are many studies comparing scalpel versus stapler without a clear advantage or disadvantage for any particular method. The comparisons within and across studies are often confounded by other technical aspects discussed later are not always controlled.

Stapler types include GIA and TA, single and multi-fire, and varying staple height from 1.0 to 2.5 mm with 2 to 6 rows of staples. A soft pancreas is considered more amenable to stapler division. Kawai et al., [21] studied the effect of pancreatic thickness on stapler efficacy finding 12 mm as a cutoff. Other groups adjust the staple height to accommodate the size and others exclude patients with a firm pancreas from the staple group. Compressing the gland before firing the stapler, closing the stapler slowly, and holding the device shut for a longer time have been suggested to lower the incidence of POPF [21-26].

Energy devices include unipolar and bipolar cautery, ultrasonic/ harmonic scalpel, and a high-energy radiowave device which all coagulate, seal, and cut. The small trials for these instruments have shown them to be safe alternatives but without a clear influence on POPF rate or other advantage [21, 27-29].

5.3. Reinforcement

The pancreatic stump exposes the transected main pancreatic duct (PD) as well as smaller pancreatic ducts, all of which can contribute to a pancreatic leak or fistula. Many methods have been explored to reinforce the cut edge to decrease the number of POPF. Direct ligation with silk or slowly absorbing monofilament suture of the main pancreatic duct is often performed when the duct can be identified regardless of the method of pancreatic division [26]. PD ligation is one of the more consistent maneuvers which decreases POPF [7].

5.3.1. Oversewing

After scalpel division, the stump is often oversewn to compress and target the smaller ducts. Slowly absorbing monofilament is generally used with either individual or running stitches; mattress sutures are common [24, 26]. Although direct ligation of the transected duct would seem to reduce POPF and has been widely recommended, there is little comparative evidence to demonstrate its utility. However, limited data would suggest that the use of a non-absorbable suture should be avoided in closure of the pancreatic stump.

5.3.2. Fibrin

The coagulation factor fibrin can be employed in a number of ways to reinforce the transected pancreas although compelling evidence of its efficacy is lacking. It is available in multiple formulations allowing for spraying, injecting, and overlaying a patch including Tisseel (Baxter International Inc.), FloSeal (Baxter International Inc.), Evicel (Ethicon), TachoSil (Nycomed Pharma), Barillas P (CSL Behring), Thrombin-JMI (King Pharmaceuticals), Quixil (Omrix Biopharmaceuticals S. A. – Ethicon) [30].

Randomized controlled trials have been performed with favorable but not consistent results. In a small study, after scalpel division, duct ligation, and suture reinforcement, half of the patients received fibrin spray treatment which decreased the POPF rate from 40% to 15% [31]. Comparing application of fibrin spray after scalpel division and duct ligation either as a simple spray application versus when followed by suture compression forming a "fibrin sandwich," the sandwich group had a significant reduction in POPF (27% to 9%) [32]. Suc et al., [33] injected fibrin into the pancreatic duct which did not influence the POPF rate. TachoSil, an absorbable collagen fleece coated with fibrinogen and thrombin available in Europe was used in two RCTs buttressing either scalpel or stapler divided stumps and did not affect POPF rate [34, 35].

5.3.3. Mesh

Meshes of various biochemical compositions can be secured over the cut end and some studies have shown promising results in decreasing POPF. Vicryl mesh, a polyglactin polymer available from Ethicon, was shown to be safe and effective with no grade B/C fistulae in a group of 26 patients after scalpel division [36]. Polyglycolic acid (PGA) mesh is a bioabsorbable synthetic polymer with cellulose-like structure which significantly decreased the rate of clinical fistulae after stapler division/reinforcement [37].

5.3.4. Intraductal Injection

Intraductal fibrin injection described above was designed to transiently obstruct the duct. Alternatively, a prolamine injection was administered in 51 patients who did not develop any POPF. The authors note that the substance was sometimes seen to extravasate from the cut edge or smaller ducts and hypothesized that the application was successful for addressing both the main and any branch ducts.

5.3.5. Biologic Patches

Biologic patches can be employed to reinforce the pancreatic stump and to provide a barrier between the pancreas and underlying vessels.

Neighboring available structures that have been reported on are the omentum, round ligament of the liver, and a seromuscular jejunal layer. In a randomized controlled trial, there was minimal improvement in POPF after the round ligament was mobilized, introduced to the pancreatic stump through a defect created in the lesser omentum and then secured in place [38]. The jejunum was used as a patch by securing the stapler-divided, PD ligated stump to a loop of jejunum with interrupted seromuscular sutures after mobilization of the duodenojejunal flexure without opening the enteric lumen. There was no improvement in the POPF rate [39].

5.3.6. Pancreaticoenteric Anastomoses

Pancreaticoenteric anastomosis is sometimes employed during reoperation for pancreatic fistula so it was hypothesized that a preemptive anastomosis during the initial operation would be effective. Two randomized controlled trials have been performed that fail to show a significant decrease in POPF from a more standard approach. A pancreaticojejunostomy in which the first jejunal loop was used for an anastomosis and for a seromuscular parenchymal patch was trialed in 136 patients dividing the patients between anastomosis and stapler division/reinforcement [40]. Pancreaticogastrostomy in comparison to ultrasonic division with ductal ligation and suture reinforcement also did not show improvement [41].

5.4. Spleen-Preserving Distal Pancreatectomy

Distal pancreatectomy can be performed removing the spleen en bloc or leaving the spleen in situ to receive its blood supply via the short gastric arteries. In a retrospective study, Goh et al., found that 0/21 patients versus 14/117 experienced grade B/C POPF after a spleen-preserving procedure [42]. Other retrospective studies have shown no difference in the rate of fistula formation [14, 15].

5.5. Preoperative Endoscopic Adjuncts

Suspecting the intact Sphincter of Oddi to be a major contributor to increased pancreatic ductal pressure and resultant fistulization, preoperative endoscopic intervention has been trialed. These maneuvers have been directed at endoscopic measures to reduce the pressure gradient across the sphincter of Oddi and therefore reduce the pressure within the main pancreatic duct.

5.5.1. Botox Injection

Temporary paralysis of the Sphincter of Oddi could allow for ductal decompression during the postoperative period. A small German trial of preoperative Sphincter of Oddi Botox administration injected 100 units of Botox into the sphincter of Oddi 0-10 days before the operation. None of the 24 patients who were able to undergo their scheduled resection experienced a grade B/C fistula or any endoscopic intervention [43].

5.5.2. Stent Placement

In a randomized controlled trial for patients with planned distal pancreatectomy, 58 patients were divided into a control group compared to endoscopic stent placement into the pancreatic duct proximal to the pancreatic parenchymal transection site. The patients who underwent endoscopic stent placement had the stent placed at the time of the laparotomy with the endoscopist and surgeon working together to place the 5 or 7 Fr stent near but not within the planned stapled transection line. There were no endoscopic complications but also no reduction in POPF rate. The POPF that occurred in the intervention arm was attributed to stent migration [44].

6. Perioperative Drain Placement

Drain placement and management varies widely between surgical practices. A drain is necessary to diagnose a biochemical leak or POPF in order to sample the amylase content. A biochemical leak, in fact, requires a surgical drain as any intervention to place a drain postoperatively would upgrade it to a grade B fistula.

6.1. Prophylactic Surgical Drainage

Surgical drains are often placed near the pancreatic stump. Closed suction is most often encountered, either a Jackson-Pratt or a Blake drain of 12 to 15 French. Some surgeons argue against routine drainage because a closed suction drain promotes fistulization, may introduce infection to a sterile fluid collection, increases one's leak rate without clinical consequence, and many patients still require additional drain placement. While the other side points out that a controlled, self-limiting pancreatic leak is better than an undrained collection with a delayed diagnosis and intervention.

A major randomized controlled trial in 2001 included both pancreaticoduodenectomy and distal pancreatectomy and showed that prophylactic surgical drainage did not improve the rate or grade of POPF. 40 of the total patients underwent distal pancreatectomy with 15 receiving a right and a left upper quadrant drain, although the positions were described in relation to the anastomoses of the pancreaticoduodenectomy patients. Subsequent analysis did not delineate the type of surgery but did show equivalence between the groups. There was no difference in in-hospital mortality, intraabdominal abscess, total number of complications, or even length of stay. 13% of patients with surgical drains still needed an interventional radiology procedure. The most common IR procedure was a drain placement for abscess, fluid collection, or hemorrhage, but also included retained drain and 2 inferior vena caval filter. They concluded that routine drain placement is not beneficial after pancreatic surgery [45].

More recently, a randomized controlled trial was conducted for just patients undergoing distal pancreatectomy acknowledging the different profile of complications. 344 patients were included divided into groups with and without routine drainage that were randomized for pancreatic texture and surgical approach. Primary outcome was any grade 2 or higher complication. There was no statistical difference between the groups for complications overall or clinically relevant pancreatic fistula. There were 2 deaths in the no drain group, both of which did develop a pancreatic fistula which was suggested to have contribute to their deaths by delay in drainage. Thus, their conclusion is that routine drainage is not absolutely necessary but due to the seriousness of the complications of no drainage, it is understandable if some surgeons continue to routinely place drains [46].

A more nontraditional suggestion was posited by Sugiyama et al., after a retrospective cohort study showed improved outcomes for drain fixation. Fixation of the drainage tip to nearby retroperitoneal tissue with a loose loop of absorbable suture decreased the number of additional postoperative procedures required and did not interfere with drain removal [47].

The available trials suggest that routine surgical drainage is not required for distal pancreatectomy. However, while trials may randomize for pancreatic texture, it has not been independently explored or discussed in a subgroup analysis.

7. Postoperative Management

7.1. Postoperative Minimally Invasive Drain Placement

The first step in stable patients with undrained or inadequately drained peripancreatic fluid collections suspicious for POPF is drainage. Postoperatively, drains can be placed minimally invasively by interventional radiology using CT or ultrasound guidance. In a retrospective analysis of 365 patients requiring IR drain placement after distal pancreatectomy, it was shown to be effective in the majority of cases and identified risk factors for the need for reoperation. The fluid collections were 2.3 to 16 cm, averaging 7.3 cm; presumably smaller collections did not require drainage and any critically ill patients requiring drainage were operatively drained. Drains were placed between post-operative days 2 and 120 (median of 23.5 days) and were in place for 3 to

220 days (median 40 days). 95% of the drains effectively drained the collection so that no reoperation was required. 40% needed readjustment or upsizing and the need for secondary manipulation was a risk factor in needing a reoperation. The authors emphasized the need for placement of the largest caliber of drain possible [10].

Any intervention or deviation from the expected clinical course, by definition, redefines a pancreatic leak to be a grade B or C fistula which can include the following treatment strategies in addition to drain placement.

7.2. Somatostatin Analogue

Somatostatin is a potent inhibitor of pancreatic secretions thus making it a promising target for drug therapy in the treatment of pancreatic leak. Several trials have been conducted assessing its use in routine post-operative management to prevent fistula formation. Its use as a treatment for diagnosed leaks is widely accepted although direct evidence of the effect on decreased drainage and any associated morbidity and length of stay is lacking. Administration is contraindicated in hyperglycemic patients as somatostatin also inhibits insulin. Side effects are most commonly gastrointestinal: nausea, vomiting, diarrhea, and abdominal pain [48].

The randomized controlled trials which address prophylactic use of octreotide center on pancreaticoduodenectomy with distal pancreatectomy as an exclusion criteria or a minor component of the whole. While some European studies showed some improvement in the POPF rate, two influential RCTs which argue against routine usage are from 1997 and 2000. In 1997, 120 patients undergoing pancreaticoduodenectomy for cancer were randomized between no octreotide and 150ug of subcutaneous octreotide every eight hours for the first five postoperative days. The octreotide group had a 12% rate of POPF vs 6% for the control group and the difference was not significant [49]. A similar negative result was seen in 2000 for pancreaticoduodenectomy patients receiving 250ug of octreotide versus placebo every eight hours for five days. Bilimoria et al., retrospectively examined patients who had distal pancreatectomy only for multiple factors including administration of prophylactic octreotide. 62 patients received 100ug to 300ug of octreotide given at the same interval. 18% of octreotide patients had a leak versus 30% of the control group but the difference was not statistically significant [7].

Octreotide was the first available somatostatin analogue. Vapreotide and Pasirotide are newer, longer-acting, more potent substitutes. In a randomized controlled trial of vapreotide given routinely after pancreatic resection every 12 hours for seven days, there was no decrease in POPF or related conditions. 52 of the 275 patients had undergone distal pancreatectomy [50]. Pasireotide is also dosed twice daily and was given for 7 days in the 2014 randomized placebo-controlled trial. Of the 539 pancreatic resection patients, 80 underwent distal pancreatectomy performed with a variety of division and reinforcement techniques. 17% of the total patients receiving Pasireotide withdrew for nausea. Notably, there was a statistically significant decrease in POPF from 17% to 8%. Length of stay was also impacted; median LOS was one day shorter with administration of the drug [48]. Subsequent cost analysis questioned the impact of the improvement in rate and length of stay but ultimately found that despite the high cost of the drug, the cost savings for interventions and daily hospitalization supported the routine use of prophylactic Pasireotide [51].

7.3. Dietary Management

Classically, patients with suspected or confirmed pancreatic leaks would be made NPO in order to disrupt the gastropancreatic neurohormonal signaling. A more modern approach encourages oral nutrition whenever tolerated.

7.3.1. Oral Nutrition

In a small subgroup analysis within a retrospective study, patients with low output pancreatic fistulae were observed to spontaneously close with no improvement when receiving parenteral nutrition [1]. A randomized controlled trial comparing the treatment of POPF after any pancreatic resection with parenteral nutrition until resolution of the fistula versus enteral nutrition through an endoscopically nasojejunal tube showed an advantage for the enteral nutrition [52]. In a group of post-distal pancreatectomy patients with POPF, patients were randomized between parenteral nutrition and oral nutrition. Oral nutrition was well tolerated and was not associated with increased length of stay or other complications [53].

7.3.2. Fluid Restriction

When 330 patients undergoing pancreatic resection (96 distal pancreatectomy) were randomized between a liberal and restricted fluid management plan, there was no advantage or disadvantage between the two groups. The liberal arm delivered a standard maintenance fluid rate of 12ml/kg/hr with 250ml boluses for urine output below 0.5ml/kg/hr. The restricted arm delivered half of that rate with boluses for low urine below 0.25ml/kg/hr. There was no effect on POPF rate although there was a slight decrease in the rate of delayed gastric emptying. Two patients did develop chronic renal failure but the rate was equal between the study arms and was attributed to related POPF [54].

7.4. Endoscopic Intervention

Preoperative endoscopic Botox injection and stent placement were previously discussed. There is also a role for post-operative POPF management again suspecting the Sphincter of Oddi to be a major contributor to the increased intraductal pressure and fistulization. Goasguen et al. reported overall success in treatment of prolonged POPF with endoscopic pancreatic sphincterotomy. Of the total 10 patients, 6 had undergone distal pancreatectomy and had a POPF diagnosed between postoperative day 3 and 21. 23 to 106 days after diagnosis, endoscopic sphincterotomy with or without stent placement was performed with successful POPF resolution 1-12 days post procedure [55].

Conclusion

The risk of pancreatic fistula formation after distal pancreatectomy is considerable by any definition of POPF. Review of the literature for the lowest risk surgical technique is confounded by the inter-trial variability in all of the many factors. The inability to compare outcomes across hospitals limits the application of some research conclusions. While there is not a single tool or pharmacological agent that can substantially decrease the rate of POPF, early postoperative recognition in those patients at higher risk may limit the clinical consequence.

References

[1] Sheehan, M. K., et al., Distal pancreatectomy: does the method of closure influence fistula formation? *Am Surg*, 2002. 68(3): p. 264-7; discussion 267-8.

[2] Yeo, C. J., et al., Six hundred fifty consecutive pancreatic-oduodenectomies in the 1990s: pathology, complications, and outcomes. *Ann Surg,* 1997. 226(3): p. 248-57; discussion 257-60.

[3] Jimenez, R. E. and Hawkins, W. G. Emerging strategies to prevent the development of pancreatic fistula after distal pancreatectomy. *Surgery,* 2012. 152(3 Suppl 1): p. S64-70.

[4] Eshmuminov, D., et al., Systematic review and meta-analysis of postoperative pancreatic fistula rates using the updated 2016 *International Study Group Pancreatic Fistula definition in patients undergoing pancreatic resection with soft and hard pancreatic texture.* HPB (Oxford), 2018.

[5] Bassi, C., et al., Postoperative pancreatic fistula: an international study group (ISGPF) definition. *Surgery*, 2005. 138(1): p. 8-13.

[6] Bassi, C., et al., The 2016 update of the International Study Group (ISGPS) definition and grading of postoperative pancreatic fistula: 11 Years After. *Surgery*, 2017. 161(3): p. 584-591.

[7] Bilimoria, M. M., et al., Pancreatic leak after left pancreatectomy is reduced following main pancreatic duct ligation. *Br J Surg*, 2003. 90(2): p. 190-6.

[8] Liang, S., Hameed, U. and Jayaraman, S. Laparoscopic pancreatectomy: indications and outcomes. *World J Gastroenterol*, 2014. 20(39): p. 14246-54.

[9] Vin, Y., et al., Management and outcomes of postpancreatectomy fistula, leak, and abscess: results of 908 patients resected at a single institution between 2000 and 2005. *J Am Coll Surg*, 2008. 207(4): p. 490-8.

[10] Cronin, C. G., et al., Interventional radiology in the management of abdominal collections after distal pancreatectomy: a retrospective review. *AJR Am J Roentgenol*, 2011. 197(1): p. 241-6.

[11] Sahakyan, M. A., et al., Laparoscopic distal pancreatectomy for pancreatic ductal adenocarcinoma: Long-term oncologic outcomes after standard resection. *Surgery,* 2017. 162(4): p. 802-811.

[12] Goh, B. K., et al., Critical appraisal of 232 consecutive distal pancreatectomies with emphasis on risk factors, outcome, and management of the postoperative pancreatic fistula: a 21-year experience at a single institution. *Arch Surg*, 2008. 143(10): p. 956-65.

[13] Seeliger, H., et al., Risk factors for surgical complications in distal pancreatectomy. *Am J Surg*, 2010. 200(3): p. 311-7.

[14] Fahy, B. N., et al., Morbidity, mortality, and technical factors of distal pancreatectomy. *Am J Surg*, 2002. 183(3): p. 237-41.

[15] Jutric, Z., et al., Preoperative computed tomography scan to predict pancreatic fistula after distal pancreatectomy using gland and tumor characteristics. *Am J Surg*, 2016. 211(5): p. 871-6.

[16] Sierzega, M., et al., Nutritional status affects the rate of pancreatic fistula after distal pancreatectomy: a multivariate analysis of 132 patients. *J Am Coll Surg*, 2007. 205(1): p. 52-9.

[17] Daouadi, M., et al., Robot-assisted minimally invasive distal pancreatectomy is superior to the laparoscopic technique. *Ann Surg,* 2013. 257(1): p. 128-32.

[18] de Rooij, T., et al., Single-Surgeon Learning Curve in 111 Laparoscopic Distal Pancreatectomies: Does Operative Time Tell the Whole Story? *J Am Coll Surg*, 2017. 224(5): p. 826-832.e1.

[19] Klompmaker, S., et al., Nationwide Evaluation of Patient Selection for Minimally Invasive Distal Pancreatectomy Using American College of Surgeons' National Quality Improvement Program. *Ann Surg,* 2017. 266(6): p. 1055-1061.

[20] Magge, D., et al., Comparative effectiveness of minimally invasive and open distal pancreatectomy for ductal adenocarcinoma. *JAMA Surg,* 2013. 148(6): p. 525-31.

[21] Kawai, M., et al., Stump closure of a thick pancreas using stapler closure increases pancreatic fistula after distal pancreatectomy. *Am J Surg,* 2013. 206(3): p. 352-9.

[22] Kajiyama, Y., et al., Quick and simple distal pancreatectomy using the GIA stapler: report of 35 cases. *Br J Surg*, 1996. 83(12): p. 1711.

[23] Misawa, T., et al., Safe and quick distal pancreatectomy using a staggered six-row stapler. *Am J Surg*, 2008. 195(1): p. 115-8.

[24] Diener, M. K., et al., DISPACT trial: a randomized controlled trial to compare two different surgical techniques of DIStal PAnCrea-Tectomy - study rationale and design. *Clin Trials*, 2008. 5(5): p. 534-45.

[25] Diener, M. K., et al., Efficacy of stapler versus hand-sewn closure after distal pancreatectomy (DISPACT): a randomised, controlled multicentre trial. *Lancet,* 2011. 377(9776): p. 1514-22.

[26] Knaebel, H. P., et al., Systematic review and meta-analysis of technique for closure of the pancreatic remnant after distal pancreatectomy. *Br J Surg,* 2005. 92(5): p. 539-46.

[27] Sugo, H., et al., Distal pancreatectomy using the harmonic scalpel. *Surgery,* 2000. 128(3): p. 490-1.

[28] Suzuki, Y., et al., Randomized clinical trial of ultrasonic dissector or conventional division in distal pancreatectomy for non-fibrotic pancreas. *Br J Surg,* 1999. 86(5): p. 608-11.

[29] Fronza, J. S., et al., Laparoscopic distal pancreatectomy using radiofrequency energy. *Am J Surg,* 2010. 199(3): p. 401-4; discussion 404.

[30] Fingerhut, A., et al., Use of sealants in pancreatic surgery: critical appraisal of the literature. *Dig Surg*, 2009. 26(1): p. 7-14.

[31] Suzuki, Y., et al., Fibrin glue sealing for the prevention of pancreatic fistulas following distal pancreatectomy. *Arch Surg*, 1995. 130(9): p. 952-5.

[32] Ohwada, S., et al., Fibrin glue sandwich prevents pancreatic fistula following distal pancreatectomy. *World J Surg*, 1998. 22(5): p. 494-8.

[33] Suc, B., et al., Temporary fibrin glue occlusion of the main pancreatic duct in the prevention of intra-abdominal complications after pancreatic resection: prospective randomized trial. *Ann Surg,* 2003. 237(1): p. 57-65.

[34] Montorsi, M., et al., Efficacy of an absorbable fibrin sealant patch (TachoSil) after distal pancreatectomy: a multicenter, randomized, controlled trial. *Ann Surg*, 2012. 256(5): p. 853-9; discussion 859-60.

[35] Sa Cunha, A., et al., Stump closure reinforcement with absorbable fibrin collagen sealant sponge (TachoSil) does not prevent pancreatic fistula after distal pancreatectomy: the FIABLE multicenter controlled randomized study. *Am J Surg*, 2015. 210(4): p. 739-48.

[36] Matsumoto, I., et al., Transpancreatic Mattress Suture with Vicryl Mesh Around the Stump During Distal Pancreatectomy: A Novel Technique for Preventing Postoperative Pancreatic Fistula. *J Am Coll Surg*, 2016. 223(2): p. e1-5.

[37] Jang, J. Y., et al., Effect of Polyglycolic Acid Mesh for Prevention of Pancreatic Fistula Following Distal Pancreatectomy: A Randomized Clinical Trial. *JAMA Surg*, 2017. 152(2): p. 150-155.

[38] Hassenpflug, M., et al., Teres Ligament Patch Reduces Relevant Morbidity After Distal Pancreatectomy (the DISCOVER Randomized Controlled Trial). *Ann Surg*, 2016. 264(5): p. 723-730.

[39] Olah, A., et al., Randomized clinical trial of techniques for closure of the pancreatic remnant following distal pancreatectomy. *Br J Surg,* 2009. 96(6): p. 602-7.

[40] Kawai, M., et al., Randomized Controlled Trial of Pancreaticojejunostomy versus Stapler Closure of the Pancreatic Stump During Distal Pancreatectomy to Reduce Pancreatic Fistula. *Ann Surg*, 2016. 264(1): p. 180-7.

[41] Sudo, T., et al., Distal pancreatectomy with duct-to-mucosa pancreaticogastrostomy: a novel technique for preventing postoperative pancreatic fistula. *Am J Surg*, 2011. 202(1): p. 77-81.

[42] Goh, B. K., Re: Distal pancreatectomy: risk factors for surgical failure in 302 consecutive cases. *Ann Surg*, 2008. 247(2): p. 392-3; author reply 393.

[43] Hackert, T., et al., Sphincter of Oddi botulinum toxin injection to prevent pancreatic fistula after distal pancreatectomy. *Surgery,* 2017. 161(5): p. 1444-1450.

[44] Frozanpor, F., et al., The effect of prophylactic transpapillary pancreatic stent insertion on clinically significant leak rate following distal pancreatectomy: results of a prospective controlled clinical trial. *Ann Surg*, 2012. 255(6): p. 1032-6.

[45] Conlon, K. C., et al., Prospective randomized clinical trial of the value of intraperitoneal drainage after pancreatic resection. *Ann Surg,* 2001. 234(4): p. 487-93; discussion 493-4.

[46] Van Buren, G., 2nd, et al., A Prospective Randomized Multicenter Trial of Distal Pancreatectomy with and Without Routine Intraperitoneal Drainage. *Ann Surg*, 2017. 266(3): p. 421-431.

[47] Sugiyama, M., et al., Secure placement of a peripancreatic drain after a distal pancreatectomy. *Am J Surg*, 2010. 199(2): p. 178-82.

[48] Allen, P. J., et al., Pasireotide for postoperative pancreatic fistula. *N Engl J Med*, 2014. 370(21): p. 2014-22.

[49] Lowy, A. M., et al., Prospective, randomized trial of octreotide to prevent pancreatic fistula after pancreaticoduodenectomy for malignant disease. *Ann Surg*, 1997. 226(5): p. 632-41.

[50] Sarr, M. G., The potent somatostatin analogue vapreotide does not decrease pancreas-specific complications after elective pancreatectomy: a prospective, multicenter, double-blinded, randomized, placebo-controlled trial. *J Am Coll Surg*, 2003. 196(4): p. 556-64; discussion 564-5; author reply 565.

[51] Ma, L. W., et al., The Cost of Postoperative Pancreatic Fistula Versus the Cost of Pasireotide: Results from a Prospective Randomized Trial. *Ann Surg*, 2017. 265(1): p. 11-16.

[52] Klek, S., et al., Enteral and parenteral nutrition in the conservative treatment of pancreatic fistula: a randomized clinical trial. *Gastroenterology*, 2011. 141(1): p. 157-63, 163.e1.

[53] Fujii, T., et al., Oral Food Intake Versus Fasting on Postoperative Pancreatic Fistula After Distal Pancreatectomy: A Multi-Institutional Randomized Controlled Trial. *Medicine (Baltimore),* 2015. 94(52): p. e2398.

[54] Grant, F., et al., Prospective Randomized Controlled Trial of Liberal Vs Restricted Perioperative Fluid Management in Patients Undergoing Pancreatectomy. *Ann Surg*, 2016. 264(4): p. 591-8.

[55] Goasguen, N., et al., Endoscopic management of pancreatic fistula after distal pancreatectomy and enucleation. *Am J Surg*, 2009. 197(6): p. 715-20.

In: Handbook of Surgical Procedures
Editor: Heather Gilbert
ISBN: 978-1-53614-580-9

Chapter 5

The Role of Endoscopic Sinus Surgery in Pediatric Patients with Cystic Fibrosis

Marco Berlucchi[1,*], Vittorio Rampinelli[2], Marco Ferrari[2], Piercarlo Poli[3], Luigi Fomasi[3], Silviana Timpano[3] and Rita Padoan[3]

[1]Department of Pediatric Otorhinolaryngology,
Spedali Civili di Brescia, Brescia, Italy
[2]Department of Otorhinolaryngology,
University of Brescia, Brescia, Italy
[3]Unit of Cystic Fibrosis, Department of Pediatric,
University of Brescia, Brescia, Italy

Abstract

Cystic fibrosis (CF) is the most common life threatening autosomal recessive disorder affecting Caucasians. Molecular genetic mutations in the CF transmembrane conductance regulator (CFTR) gene alter function

* Corresponding Author Email: marco.berlucchi@tin.it.

of CFTR protein, which leads to dysfunction in chloride channel on epithelial surface of exocrine glands. In the head and neck area, the pathology involves mostly paranasal sinuses starting from childhood. Chronic and recurrent rhinosinusitis with or without nasal polyposis and mucocele of sinuses are the main disorders observed in CF patients. About 20-25% of these patients will require sinus surgery. Regarding surgical treatment, endoscopic sinus surgery (ESS) for management of paranasal sinus diseases in CF patients is undoubtedly a challenge for the surgeon. Moreover, evidence-based guidelines regarding the precise indications for surgery are currently lacking. Even if ESS is undeniably needed for management of sinonasal complications and can improve CF-related nasal symptoms, its role with regards to timing of surgery and consequent improvement of pulmonary function is not well described. Moreover, underlying medical issues such as acquired coagulopathies and advanced pulmonary disease, raise perioperative morbidity in these patients, with consequent and prolonged hospitalization. Indeed, the surgeon is often faced with distorted anatomy, due to anomalous development of nasal and paranasal structures or multiple revision operations. Therefore, multidisciplinary management of paranasal sinus disease in patients affected by CF is pivotal to achieve the correct surgical indication, prepare the patient for surgery, and address possible perioperative complications. The authors describe the indications of ESS in CF patients, analyzing personal experience in the diagnosis and treatment of CF-related sinus disorders. Finally, data on follow-up after ESS, pulmonary function, and nutritional status will be presented.

INTRODUCTION

Cystic fibrosis (CF) is the most common life-threatening autosomal recessive genetic disease in the Caucasian population, and it is estimated that over 100,000 worldwide are affected. Thanks to advances in CF therapies, overall survival has increased. At present, more than 50% of those affected reach adulthood in USA, Europe, and Australia [1, 2].

CF is a multiorgan disease, with morbidity and mortality determined in the great majority of cases by progressive respiratory failure. As for the lower airways, at the basis of sinonasal manifestations there is a functional defect in the cystic fibrosis transmembrane conductance regulator (CFTR) gene, located on the long arm of chromosome 7. This gene encodes for a protein expressed on the epithelium of the airways where it works as a channel for chloride and bicarbonate and a regulator of other ion transport channels. The imbalance between ion transport channels (low Cl^- secretion, Na^+ hyper-reabsorption, reduced pH of airway surface liquid due to defective HCO_3^- secretion) lead to airway surface dehydration, causing thick and viscous secretions, chronic infections, and inflammation.

Generally, the clinician and the multidisciplinary team that deals with the treatment of the patient focus on lung disease, which, due to its characteristics, is the most fearsome manifestation. For this reason, the sinonasal manifestations of the disease are often underdiagnosed and not adequately treated. The patient himself, when the symptoms of the manifestation appear, may not give them an adequate relevance or do not have a wellness status as a comparison in case of an event that has always been present, and does not report symptoms to the clinician.

To date, the relationship between sinonasal manifestations and pulmonary disease has not been fully elucidated and there are several interesting theories that correlate aggravation of sinonasal status with a worsening of lung function, even after lung transplantation. However, it is certain that sinonasal symptomatology worsens the patient's quality of life, and therefore manifestations of the upper airways must be sought by the clinician through correct medical history, also considering the underestimations referred by the patient.

To date, considerable progress has been made in medical and surgical treatment of ENT pathologies in CF, and it is now possible to successfully treat such manifestations and improve the patient's quality of life.

In CF patients, a clinical picture of chronic/recurrent rhinosinusitis is generally observed and may be associated or not with nasal polyps. Moreover, a mucocele of sinus can develop in some patients. Another characteristic of sinonasal involvement is hypoplasia/aplasia of some paranasal sinuses that is usually found at imaging.

PHYSIOPATHOLOGY

In the sinonasal epithelium there are two layers of liquid with different densities. A first fluid delineates and wets the eyelashes and is low in density, while the second is represented by a layer of high-density, superficial mucus that has the function of trapping inhaled particles and transporting them through coordinated ciliary beat in the digestive tract [3]. This mechanism is called mucociliary clearance and is obviously an innate defense mechanism, guarding the upper (and inferior) airways.

The mechanisms of mucociliary clearance in the patient with CF are dysfunctional; due to altered anionic transport of mutated CFTR, there is a noticeable change in the viscoelastic properties of mucus, with increase in viscosity from 30 to 60 times above normal: the dense secretions obstruct the sinus ostia and create a state of hypoxia with edema and secondary ciliary dyskinesia; obviously this scenario facilitates bacterial colonization.

Bacteria release many substances that reduce the frequency of ciliary beats and help to create a chronic inflammatory state, promoting hyperplasia of mucus producing cells, along with squamous metaplasia and loss of cilia. Macroscopically, all these effects lead to stasis of infected mucus, inflammation, and alteration of gas exchange. The increase in $PaCO_2$ that is established also promotes edema and decreases mucus ciliary clearance [4].

In this complex pathogenic picture, anatomical anomalies, nasal polyposis, and mucoceles can be found.

ALTERATION OF THE ANATOMY OF THE PARANASAL SINUSES

In recent years, the use of CT has been widely used pre-operatively to evaluate the anatomy of the sinonasal tract of patients with CF.

An often-observed feature is the lack of development or hypoplasia of the frontal and sphenoid sinuses. These sinuses develop mainly in the post-natal period and the pathogenic mechanisms underlying CF somehow hinder their normal development [5]. The same mechanisms are also be responsible for reduced postnatal growth of the sinuses present at birth (maxillary and ethmoid).

It is hypothesized that chronic inflammatory status and reduced ventilation that reduce pneumatization are at the basis of this alteration. This hypothesis is supported by the fact that in the course of chronic otitis media there is no pneumatization of the mastoid.

Another possible finding is demineralization of bone walls, and in particular the medial wall of the maxillary sinus (which can also be medialized). It is also important to underline that a bone demineralization framework with medialization of the medial wall of the maxillary sinus is strongly suggestive for mucocele.

Nasal Polyposis

CF patients have a high incidence of nasal polyposis associated with chronic rhinosinusitis, which is present in up to 48% of patients [6]. On the contrary, in the child without CF nasal polyposis is an extremely rare phenomenon, and in fact the finding of nasal polyposis in the pediatric age must make the clinician evoke possible previously undiagnosed CF.

Nasal polyps in non-CF patients are benign proliferations of mucosal cells, characterized histologically by edema, hyperplasia of mucus producing cells of the epithelium, thickening of the basal membrane, and the presence of numerous leucocytes, especially eosinophils (eosinophil-mediated inflammation).

CF related polyps have characteristics in common with those in the general population: focal edema, hyperplasia, atrophy or metaplasia of the epithelium, lamina propria which presents small vessels, and focal accumulations of inflammatory cells. Specific features of CF-related polyps are: thin basal membrane, lack of eosinophils, presence of neutrophil-mediated inflammation, acid mucin in the glands, continuous and fenestrated capillaries, and the presence of morphologically atypical plasma cells [7].

The physio-pathogenetic mechanisms underlying the formation of nasal polyps in CF remain unclear to date, as well as those of the healthy population. It is also not clear why some patients with polyposis have symptoms, while others remain asymptomatic.

MUCOCELE

Mucocele is a secreting mucus cyst, delineated by epithelium, which can localize and grow within a paranasal sinus with a concentric expansion [8]. It is a benign disorder, but with the accumulation of secretions it increases in size until the surrounding bone structures are moved and eroded. Thus, ocular and intracranial complications can arise. They can become infected, and in this case are referred to as mucopioceles.

Mucocele is believed to be formed due to obstruction of the sinus ostium. In the non-CF population it is typically a sinonasal adult disease, with onset generally in the third and fourth decades. The most frequently affected sinuses are the frontal and the ethmoid, and less frequently the sphenoid and maxillary [9]. It is a rare sinonasal disease in childhood, and in most cases is associated with CF. The mucocele is indeed part of the sinonasal complications typical of the disease [10], with a prevalence of up to 16% of patients with upper-airway disorders [11]. Some authors also suggest also that when the mucocele(s) is diagnosed in the first months of life, its formation had likely begun during intrauterine life [8].

The detection of mucocele in a child without a diagnosis of CF requires diagnostic investigation and a sweat test.

MICROBIOLOGY

The bacteria typically isolated from nasal material cultures of the patient with CF are *Pseudomonas aeruginosa, Staphylococcus aureus, Escherichia coli, Burkholderia cepacia, Acinetobacter* spp, *Stenotrophomonas maltophilia, Haemophilus influenzae, Streptococci,* and anaerobia.

The frequency of colonization of the lower airways by *Pseudomonas* in patients with chronic rhinosinusitis and polyposis is high; such colonization starts from the upper airways and then descends into the lower airways [12].

The association between cultures of the upper and the lower airways is verified, and has also demonstrated from a genotypical point of view: it is therefore correct to think that the paranasal sinuses can act as a reservoir for recurrent pulmonary infections in the disease [13]. It is therefore particularly important to improve the health of the sinuses as much as possible. Hence the importance of considering and actively searching for the presence of sinonasal symptoms during patient interview. Moreover, for these reasons sinonasal surgery is indicated in preparation for lung transplantation.

Clinical Manifestations

Symptomatology is due to chronic/recurrent rhinosinusitis associated with or not nasal polyposis. Patients can complain of nasal obstruction, anterior and posterior rhinorrhea, hyposmia/anosmia, headache, facial pain, and fever. Moreover, day and night oral respiration, snoring, decreased sleep quality, halitosis, changes in voice, and otalgia are other signs and symptoms that can be found.

When a mucocele is present, ocular signs and symptoms such as proptosis, epiphora, visual disturbances, and alterations of ocular motility may be observed. Mucocele can have a presentation without classical symptomatology and only with atypical manifestations. It is therefore essential not only to keep in mind the possibility of mucocele, but to seek it actively, especially in unclear and atypical situations.

Diagnosis

If sinonasal manifestations are evident on history, the patient must be undergone careful ENT assessment, and, in particular, rhinoscopy under local anesthesia must be performed. At nasal endoscopy, it is possible to identify sinonasal anatomic anomalies (i.e., nasal septum deviation, concha bullosa, hypertrophy of the inferior turbinate), pathological nasal secretions, nasal polyps (Figure 1), and bulging of the medial wall of the maxillary sinus (Figure 2) and/or anterior wall of sphenoid suspicious for mucocele.

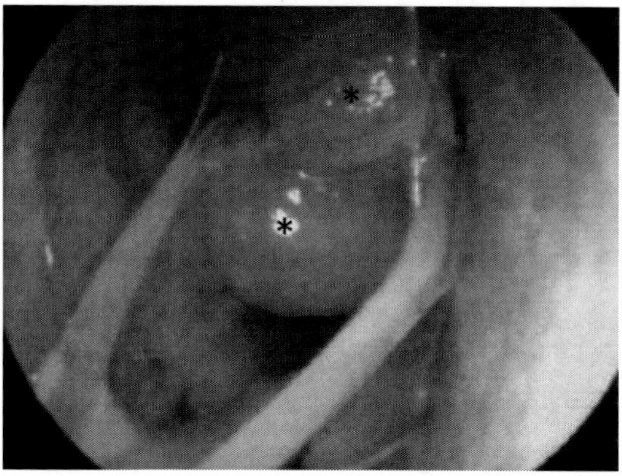

Figure 1. Nasal polyps (asterisks) associated with dense secretions completely obstructing the right nasal fossa.

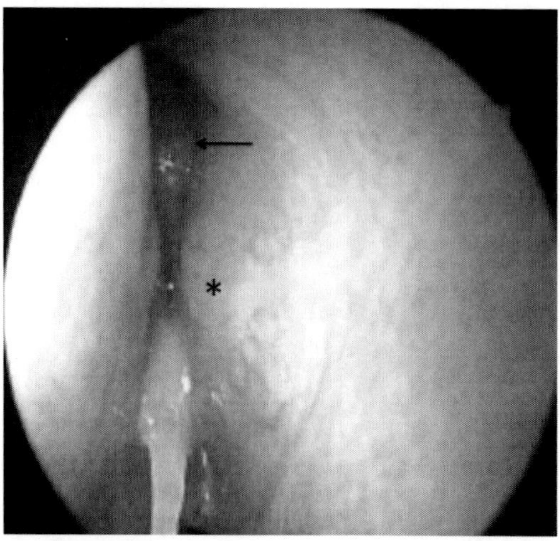

Figure 2. Bulging of the medial wall of the left maxillary sinus (asterisk). The left middle turbinate is still visible (arrow).

The next diagnostic step is represented by imaging such as CT or MR of the paranasal sinuses. These radiologic studies allow overall assessment of the patient's sinonasal anatomy, identifying the sinonasal pathology and its extension.

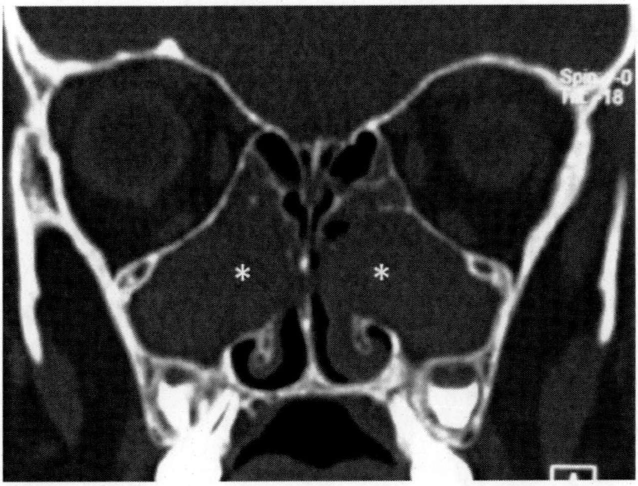

Figure 3. At coronal CT scan, a bilateral mucocele (white asterisks) of the maxillary sinus associated with erosion of its medial wall is found.

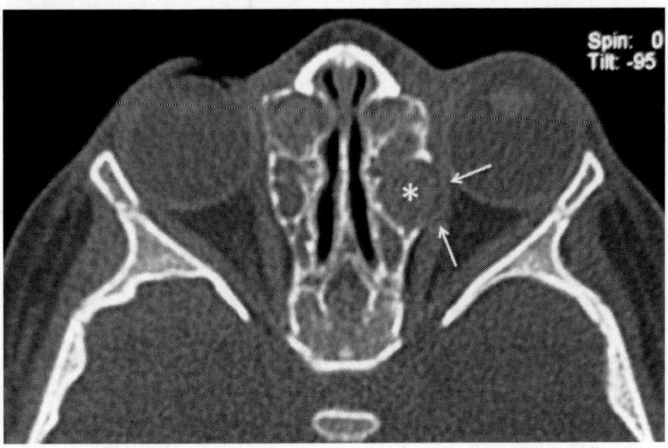

Figure 4. At axial CT scan, a left ethmoidal mucocele (white asterisk) is observed. Moreover, erosion of the lamina papyracea (white arrows) associated with displacement of the left medial rectus muscle is evident.

Usually, mucocele appears as a complete opacification of a single sinus. As the mucocele expands, it remodels the local anatomy by slowly compressing surrounding structures, with consequent resorption of the neighboring bony walls (Figure 3).

Imaging (CT and/or MR) is needed to confirm diagnosis and identify bony changes and intraorbital (Figure 4) or intracranial extension of the expansive fluid-collection(s).

Cases of bilateral maxillary mucoceles have been described, with CT showing a typical figure called "hourglass image," which is formed by bilateral mucoceles occluding nasal cavities [8].

In the literature, however, it is believed that the findings that can be visualized by imaging cannot be considered to be a reliable measure for outcomes after medical or surgical intervention. Some authors analyzed CT scans performed in patients with CF before and after surgery, graduating them with the Lund-Mackay (LM) score, and found that despite medical or surgical treatment there was no significant difference in the LM score of scans before and after intervention. Although CT is an important diagnostic step, performing multiple scans to monitor the disease is not useful and does not correlate with exacerbations of the disease or medical or surgical treatment. The study states that LM is a useful method of CT analysis, but does not provide adequate stratification for analysis of changes in opacification of the sinuses over time, especially in the case of partial opacification [14].

Although this study has not highlighted changes in CT, it underlines however that following intervention, improvements of symptomatology have been noted in the literature and hypothesizes that the benefit of surgery can be demonstrated by other parameters that analyze the quality of life [5, 15-16].

TREATMENT

In the last few decades, life expectancy of individuals suffering from cystic fibrosis (CF) has significantly improved, resulting in new medical perspectives for these patients. Life-saving treatments, indeed, have been progressively associated with interventions aimed to improve quality of life [17].

Since the sinonasal tract is involved in the majority of CF patients, otolaryngologists have a significant role in the multi-disciplinary management of these patients [17].

Management of chronic rhinosinusitis (CRS) in CF is challenging and is based on the combination of both medical and surgical therapy [18]. Appropriate medical therapy typically includes oral and/or intravenous antibiotics, topical and/or systemic steroids, and saline irrigations [19-20]. In the literature, surgery is indicated when CRS does not respond to conservative maximal medical therapy and is performed in 20–60% of patients with CF [21-23]. This variable frequency of surgically treated patients mirrors the absence of consensus on indications and timing for surgery. In fact, no universally accepted guidelines for the surgical management of CRS in CF-patients are available.

Despite the large number of studies on this topic published during the last decade, the majority of these combined data from both adults and children, thus precluding firm conclusions on these exceedingly different groups of patients. Furthermore, only a few studies reached a good level of evidence [19-20].

The decision to indicate surgery is typically based on a combination of factors: clinical and/or radiological evidence of sinonasal disease (i.e., massive obstructive polyposis, diplopia, mucocele), patient-reported symptoms, sinusitis-related detriment of quality of life, overall health and nutrition status, occurrence of faltering growth, pulmonary conditions including recent pneumonia exacerbations and lung function parameters, patient personality, and patient-physician relationship [24, 25]. In the literature, there is conflicting evidence whether genotype correlates with severity of sinonasal disease and need for surgery. Some studies have demonstrated a relationship between homozygous F508 mutations and the degree of sinusitis, presence of polyps, and need for surgery [26-27]. Other studies, however, failed in showing an association between the homozygous F508 genotype and need for sinus surgery [17, 28].

CT and MRI definitely help in selecting patients who need surgery, depicting two clinical-radiological scenarios: 1) the most typical finding requiring surgery is the complete opacification of the nasal cavities due to massive polyposis and dense nasal secretions, with possible decalcification of the bony boundaries (i.e., ethmoidal roof, lamina papyracea); 2) other patients present with mucocele(s).

To date, 153 patients affected by CF are regularly followed at Unit of Cystic Fibrosis, Department of Pediatric, University of Brescia – Italy. Between December 2003 and May 2017, based on the aforementioned concepts, 43 (28%) of these patients underwent surgical treatment at Department of Pediatric Otorhinolaryngology, Spedali Civili di Brescia, Brescia - Italy. Thirty-seven and six children were operated for mucocele of paranasal sinus and CRS associated with massive nasal polyposis, respectively.

Surgical Notes

Historically, surgery consisted of open approaches to the sinuses (i.e., Caldwell-Luc procedure). Currently, endoscopic sinus surgery (ESS) is considered the mainstay of treatment of refractory inflammatory disease of the paranasal sinuses in CF patients. All our patients underwent such surgical conservative procedure. The key concept of ESS is widening the sinus ostia and removing obstructive nasal polyps to improve mucous drainage, provide proper ventilation of air spaces, and guarantee adequate penetration of topical medications (Figure 5).

A number of general perils of ESS are emphasized when operating CF patients. The development of the paranasal sinuses can be incomplete, thus resulting in distorted and misleading anatomical configurations that can favor disorientation of the surgeon and subsequent complications. Continuous infections and multiple operations can subvert the sinonasal anatomy, further hindering the anatomical orientation during surgery. Thinning of the bony boundaries, typically involving the lamina papyracea and skull base, can facilitate the inadvertent injury of orbital and intracranial structures. Moreover, the bony lamellae of the nasoethmoidal complex are frequently resorbed, leading to the lack of anatomical landmarks that usually guide the surgeon during dissection. Furthermore, the active inflammatory process results in massive, dense secretions and increased bleeding. All the above-mentioned factors make ESS challenging and augment the risk of surgical complications, such as orbital injury and iatrogenic cerebrospinal fluid leak.

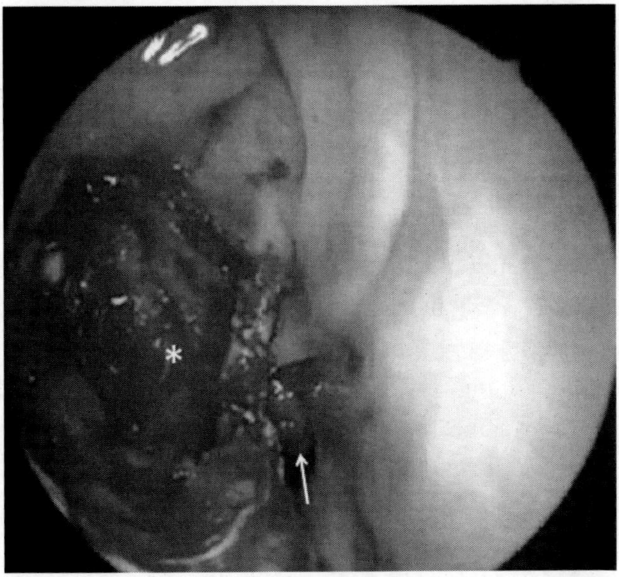

Figure 5. A right wide middle antrostomy (white asterisk) is observed at endoscopic view. Mild adenoidal hypertophy (white arrow) is present.

As an additional remark, underlying systemic alterations, such as acquired coagulopathies and advanced pulmonary disease, further raise the perioperative morbidity and lengthen hospitalization. Therefore, multidisciplinary management is of utmost importance not only to ensure the correct indications for surgery, but also to provide adequate preoperative preparation and minimize the possibility of perioperative complications. In particular, preoperative medical treatment with antibiotics and steroids associated with chest physiotherapy is mandatory to improve pulmonary function and nasal status. The surgical technique should also be customized in accordance with the physiopathology of CF: narrow and "minimalist" sinusotomies should be avoided in favor of wide and regular communications between sinuses and the nasal cavity; on the other hand, unnecessary mucosal stripping is strongly discouraged to minimize bone exposure and subsequent granulation. In line with this concept, a systematic review by Crockett et al. concluded that large maxillary antrostomies or modified medial maxillectomies provide significant improvement of the quality of life and sinus symptom scores, shorten hospitalization, and reduce the need for antibiotics [29]. By virtue of the chronic nature of CF and the necessity to recurrently manage symptoms, less invasive procedures, such as simple polypectomy, have also been proposed. However, early recurrence of nasal polyps is more likely in patients undergoing polypectomy alone than in those undergoing polypectomy associated with functional sinus surgery (ethmoidectomy and antrostomy) [30]. Balloon catheter sinuplasty has recently been introduced for the treatment of CRS in pediatric patients. It is safe and effective and has the advantage of not requiring tissue removal, thus sparing most of the sinonasal mucosal lining [31]. Consequently, although no studies on the efficacy of balloon catheter sinuplasty in patients with CF are currently available, the procedure should be considered as a promising alternative to standard ESS.

As an additional refinement, when dealing with complex, recurrent cases, a neuronavigation system may be helpful to maintain anatomical orientation and avoid dreadful complications.

Outcomes

In view of the abovementioned criticisms, ESS can be considered as a safe procedure in patients with CF when performed by expert surgeons [32].

Patients who mainly benefit from surgery are those developing CRF due to both CF and anatomic variants compromising the spontaneous ventilation of sinuses, resulting in nasal edema/polyposis and drainage obstruction.

A recent review by Liang et al. reported that sinonasal symptoms (nasal obstruction, rhinorrhea, headaches, facial pain, and olfaction impairment), which were evaluated with validated questionnaires and/or subjective reports, invariably improve following sinus surgery [19]. Accordingly, improvement of CF-related CRS signs (polyposis, edema, mucopurulence, crusting, and/or scarring) was demonstrated in more than 50% of the included studies [19]. For instance, Virgin et al. reported significant improvement of both SNOT-22 and Lund-Kennedy score at one year after surgery [18]. Shatz et al. found a significant reduction of prescriptions for intravenous antibiotics for pneumonia after ESS [33]. However, this finding was not confirmed by other authors [34]. In fact, there is conflicting evidence whether ESS significantly modifies pulmonary outcomes in CF patients [19]. Kempainen and colleagues found no difference in number of days spent in hospital pre- and post-operatively [34]. Interestingly, patients who show the greatest sinonasal-related benefit from surgery are those with higher baseline pulmonary function: CF patients with a baseline %FEV1 above >70% predicted exhibited greater improvements in sinus symptoms after surgery than those undergoing medically alone [17].

Although several studies have recommended ESS in patients undergoing lung transplantation [33], this practice has largely lost popularity. Leung et al. demonstrated that lung allograft re-colonization occurs regardless of prior sinus surgery, concluding that prophylactic ESS is not beneficial [35].

Stringent and multidisciplinary follow-up is of paramount relevance to ensure adequate postoperative medical therapy and, ultimately, optimize surgical outcomes: ESS followed by intensive post-operative medical therapy (2 weeks of antibiotics, 6 months of nasal irrigations, and 12 months of topical nasal steroids) resulted in eradication of pathogenic sinonasal bacteria for up to 1 year [22].

It is important to highlight and counsel the patient's family that ESS does not provide a definitive cure for CF-related CRS: being a genetic, systemic disease, CF prevents normalization of sinonasal mucosa, though adequately managed.

Therefore, patients and their family should be made aware about the need to undergo multiple ESS procedures throughout their life; in fact, the revision rate for CF-related CRS ranges between 20% and 100% after a period of 2–4 years from primary surgery; this rate increases parallel to the severity of polyposis at primary presentation [36]. Intuitively, recurrence is particularly common when surgical intervention is incomplete and/or when adjunct treatment with antibiotics is inadequate.

Regarding our cohort of study, a recurrence of disease was observed in 6/6 (100%) patients who were operated for CRS associated with nasal polyposis, whereas no recurrence was found in 37 children operated for paranasal mucocele with a mean follow-up of 52 months after surgery. Finally, data about pulmonary function and nutritional status did not change after surgery (Table 1).

Table 1. Pulmonary function and nutritional status evaluated before and after ESS

	Before surgery (1 month)	**After surgery (1 month)**	**p-value**
FEV_1 % predicted value	97,2	97,9	0,7
BMI (z-score)	-0,22	-0,27	0,19

ESS: endoscopic sinus surgery.

CONCLUSION

CF is a multisystem disease, frequently involving the sinonasal tract and manifesting with recurrent CRS with or not nasal polyposis and the tendency to develop paranasal mucoceles.

Evidence-based guidelines on the surgical management of CF-related CRS are lacking. Some evidence suggests that ESS could improve nasal symptoms and is strongly recommended to manage sinonasal complications. On the other hand, the timing of surgery and its role in improvement of pulmonary function remain a controversial issue.

When it occurs, mucocele of paranasal sinus is an absolute surgical indication and ESS is considered the surgical approach of choice.

However, ESS for CF-patients is challenging because of technical complexity and unfavorable underlying medical conditions that complicate perioperative medical management.

Consequently, a multidisciplinary approach to CF patients is the pivotal strategy to ensure the adequacy of surgical indication, optimize the general status of the patient, and manage possible perioperative complications.

REFERENCES

[1] Cystic Fibrosis Foundation. Cystic Fibrosis Foundation Patient Registry Annual Data Report. *Cyst. Fibros. Found. Patient Regist* (2017). *Annu. Data Report. Bethesda* 1–15.

[2] Ahern, S., Sims, G., Esler, M., Oldroyd, J., Dean, J., Bell, S. (2016). The Australian Cystic Fibrosis Data Registry Annual Report. *Monash Univ.* 1–52.

[3] Chaaban, M.R., Kejner, A., Rowe, S.M., Woodworth, B.A. (2013). Cystic fibrosis chronic rhinosinusitis: a comprehensive review. *Am J Rhinol Allergy,* 27(5):387-95.

[4] Kang, S.H., Dalcin Pde, T., Piltcher, O.B., Migliavacca Rde, O. (2015). Chronic rhinosinusitis and nasal polyposis in cystic fibrosis: update on diagnosis and treatment. *J Bras Pneumol,* 41(1):65-76.

[5] Gysin, C., Alothman, G.A., Papsin, B.C. (2000). Sinonasal disease in cystic fibrosis: clinical characteristics, diagnosis, and management. *Pediatr Pulmonol,* 30(6):481-9.

[6] Robertson, J.M., Friedman, E.M., Rubin, B.K. (2008). Nasal and sinus disease in cystic fibrosis. *Paediatr Respir Rev,* 9(3):213-9.

[7] Beju, D., Meek, W.D., Kramer, J.C. (2004). The ultrastructure of the nasal polyps in patients with and without cystic fibrosis. *J Submicrosc Cytol Pathol,* 36(2):155-65.

[8] Di Cicco, M., Costantini, D., Padoan, R., Colombo, C. (2005). Paranasal mucoceles in children with cystic fibrosis. *Int J Pediatr Otorhinolaryngol,* 69(10):1407-13.

[9] Capra, G.G., Carbone, P.N., Mullin, D.P. (2012). Paranasal sinus mucocele. *Head Neck Pathol,* 6(3):369-72.

[10] Nicollas, R., Facon, F., Sudre-levillain, I., Forman, C., Roman, S., Triglia, J.M. (2006) Pediatric paranasal sinus mucoceles: etiologic factors, management and outcome. *Int J Pediatr Otorhinolaryngol,* 70(5):905-8.

[11] Horesh, E., Colin, A.A., Casiano, R., Wester, S.T. (2015). An atypical presentation of sinus mucopyocele in a pediatric cystic fibrosis patient. *Clin Ophthalmol,* 9:821-4.

[12] Roby, B.B., Mcnamara, J., Finkelstein, M., Sidman, J. (2008). Sinus surgery in cystic fibrosis patients: comparison of sinus and lower airway cultures. *Int J Pediatr Otorhinolaryngol,* 72(9):1365-9.

[13] Mainz, J.G., Koitschev, A. (2009). Management of chronic rhinosinusitis in CF. *J Cyst Fibros*, 8 Suppl 1:S10-4.

[14] Mcmurphy, A.B., Morriss, C., Roberts, D.B., Friedman, E,M. (2007). The usefulness of computed tomography scans in cystic fibrosis patients with chronic sinusitis. *Am J Rhinol,* 21(6):706-10.

[15] Nishioka, G.J., Cook, P.R. (1996). Paranasal sinus disease in patients with cystic fibrosis. *Otolaryngol Clin North Am,* 29(1):193-205.

[16] Yung, M.W., Gould, J., Upton, G.J. (2002). Nasal polyposis in children with cystic fibrosis: a long-term follow-up study. *Ann Otol Rhinol Laryngol,* 111(12 Pt 1):1081-6.

[17] Ayoub, N., Thamboo, A., Habib, A.R., Nayak, J.V., Hwang, P.H. (2017). Determinants and outcomes of upfront surgery versus medical therapy for chronic rhinosinusitis in cystic fibrosis. *Int Forum Allergy Rhinol,* 7(5):450-458.

[18] Virgin, F.W., Rowe, S.M., Wade, M.B., et al. (2012). Extensive surgical and comprehensive postoperative medical management for

cystic fibrosis chronic rhinosinusitis. *Am J Rhinol Allergy,* 26(1):70–75.

[19] Liang, J., Higgins, T.S., Ishman, S.L., et al. (2013). Surgical management of chronic rhinosinusitis in cystic fibrosis: a systematic review. *Int Forum Allergy Rhinol*, 3:814–822.

[20] Liang, J., Higgins, T., Ishman, S.L., et al. (2014) Medical management of chronic rhinosinusitis in cystic fibrosis: a systematic review. *Laryngoscope*, 124:1308– 1313.

[21] Mainz, JG., Schien, M., Naehrlich, L., Kading, M., Thoss, K., Frey, G., et al. (2010). Prevalence of CF- related chronic rhinosinusitis--results from a multicentre interdisciplinary study. *J Cyst Fibros,* 33rd European Cystic Fibrosis Conference p. 118 120.

[22] Aanaes, K., Rasmussen, N., Pressler, T., et al. (2012). Extensive endoscopic image-guided sinus surgery decreases BPI-ANCA in patients with cystic fibrosis. *Scand J Immunol,* 76(6):573–579.

[23] Ramsey, B., Richardson M.A. (1992). Impact of sinusitis in cystic fibrosis. *The Journal of allergy and clinical immunology,* 90(3 Pt 2):547–552.

[24] Soler, Z.M., Rudmik, L., Hwang, P.H, et al. (2013). Patient- centered decision making in the treatment of chronic rhinosinusitis. *Laryngoscope*, 123:2341–2346.

[25] Rudmik, L., Soler, Z.M., Mace, J.C., et al. (2015). Using pre-operative SNOT-22 score to inform patient decision for endoscopic sinus surgery. *Laryngoscope*, 125–1522:1517.

[26] Jorissen, M.B., De Boeck, K., Cuppens, H. (1999). Genotype-phenotype correlations for the paranasal sinuses in cystic fibrosis. *Am J Respir Crit Care Med*, 159:1412–1416.

[27] Berkhout, M.C., van Rooden, C.J., Rijintjes, E., et al. (2014). Sinonasal manifestations of cystic fibrosis: a correla- tion between genotype and phenotype? *J Cyst Fibros*, 13:442–448. 23.

[28] Do, B.A., Lands, L.C., Saint-Martin, C., et al. (2014). Effect of the F508del genotype on outcomes of endoscopic sinus surgery in children with cystic fibrosis. *Int J Pediatr Otorhinolaryngol*, 78:1133–1137.

[29] Crockett, D.J., Wilson, K.F., Meier, J.D. (2013). Perioperative strategies to improve sinus surgery outcomes in patients with cystic fibrosis: a systematic review. *Otolaryngol Head Neck Surg,* 149(1):30-9.

[30] Crockett, D.M., McGill, T.J., Healy, G.B., Friedman, E.M., Salkeld, L.J. (1987). Nasal and paranasal sinus surgery in children with cystic fibrosis. *Ann Otol Rhinol Laryngol,* 96(4):367- 72.

[31] Sedaghat, A.R., Cunningham, M.J. (2011). Does balloon catheter sinuplasty have a role in the surgical management of pediatric sinus disease? *Laryngoscope,* 121(10):2053-4.

[32] Macdonald, K.I., Gipsman, A., Magit, A., Fandino, M., Massoud, E., Witterick, I.J., et al. (2012). Endoscopic sinus surgery in patients with cystic fibrosis: a systematic review and meta-analysis of pulmonary function. *Rhinology,* 50(4):360-9.

[33] Shatz, A. (2006). Management of recurrent sinus disease in children with cystic fibrosis: a com- bined approach. *Otolaryngol Head Neck Surg,* 135: 248-252.

[34] Kempainen, R.R., Sajan, J.A., Pylkas, A.M., et al. (2012). Effect of endoscopic sinus surgery on pulmonary status of adults with cystic fibrosis. *Otolaryngol Head Neck Surg*, 147(3):557-62.

[35] Leung, M.K., Rachakonda, L., Weill, D., Hwang, P.H. (2008). Effects of sinus surgery on lung transplantation out- comes in cystic fibrosis. *Am J Rhinol*, 22:192– 196.

[36] Rickert, S., Banuchi, V.E., Germana, J.D., Stewart, M.G., April, M.M. (2010). Cystic fibrosis and endoscopic sinus surgery: Relationship between nasal polyposis and likelihood of revision endoscopic sinus surgery in patients with cystic fibrosis. *Arch Otolaryngol Head Neck Surgery,* 136 (10):988–992.

In: Handbook of Surgical Procedures
Editor: Heather Gilbert
ISBN: 978-1-53614-580-9

Chapter 6

MININVASIVE SURGICAL APPROACH IN ENDOSCOPIC SINUS SURGERY (ESS)

Federico Sireci[1], MD , Francesco Galletti[2] and Frank Rikki Canevari[3]
[1]ENT Section, ARNAS Fatebenefratelli Hospital, Palermo, Italy
[2]Department of Otorhinolaryngology, University of Messina, Italy
[3]Department of Otorhinolaryngology, Head and Neck Surgery, University of Genoa, Genoa, Italy

ABSTRACT

The minimally invasive sinus technique, (MIST) is different from minimally invasive sinus surgery. MIST implies a treatment philosophy and surgical model that is quite different from functional endoscopic sinus surgery (FESS).

The goals of this article are to discuss the origins of functional sinus surgery as it relates to the evolution of FESS and MIST, define MIST as a philosophy and surgical model, discuss treatment of surgical sinus disease, and challenge the rationale for our departure from Messerklinger's "functional" concepts into what will be referred to as "contemporary FESS." Many authors address the reduced revision rate (compared with FESS) following initial intervention with MIST, the potential to markedly reduce the rate of intranasal synechiae, and the reduction in immediate postoperative morbidity.

Keywords: minimally invasive, sinusitis, endoscopic sinus surgery

INTRODUCTION

Since its introduction in the mid-1980s, functional endoscopic sinus surgery (FESS) has become the standard surgical intervention for patients with chronic sinusitis refractory to medical therapy. In fact, FESS represented a targeted intervention, aimed at restoring normal sinus mucosal physiology as first described by Messerklinger in 1978 [1].

Through his endoscopic examination of the nose, Messerklinger describes a pattern of shifting light reflexes seen on the mucosal surface of the sinuses representing mucociliary movement that we now recognize as mucociliary transport or clearance. Using endoscopy in conjunction with time-lapse photography, he examined the direction of mucus movement and found that clearance was directed from the larger sinuses to their respective ostia. He also noted that contact between mucosal surfaces leads to disruption of mucociliary movement, thereby causing retention of secretions with subsequent obstruction of the subordinate maxillary, frontal, and anterior ethmoid sinuses. Furthermore, he recognized that contact is most likely to occur in the narrow transition spaces (i.e., ethmoidal infundibulum, hiatus semilunaris superior, and nasofrontal recess). Although contact may be a result of a number of causes, such as inflammation from environmental irritants, allergic rhinitis, viral infection, or anatomic distortions, these factors are most influential to the disruption of sinus physiology and development of sinusitis when they directly affect the aforementioned transition spaces. The theory that transition spaces represent the primary physiologic/anatomic bottleneck for the development of sinusitis is further supported by the high frequency with which the computerized tomography (CT) and clinical examination findings show inflammation limited to the maxillary, frontal, and anterior ethmoid sinuses; the posterior ethmoid and sphenoid sinuses do not drain into transition spaces.

Another critical realization in the development of FESS was that mucosal damage and mucociliary dysfunction is a reversible process. Before Messerklinger, most believed that mucosal damage found in chronic sinusitis was irreversible, and, therefore, procedures such as the Caldwell- Luc involved stripping of the sinus mucosa. In his clinical experience with more than 2,500 patients, Stammberger [2] showed that once the transition spaces are cleared of disease, the larger sinuses usually heal without being touched, even if mucosal damage seemed "almost irreversible". Recent studies examining mucociliary clearance have shown that patients with chronic sinusitis have impaired mucociliary movement and that FESS is capable of correcting mucociliary dysfunction in these patients, thus showing the reversibility of disease [3-6]. To create optimal conditions for reversal of disease to occur, surgical intervention should avoid destruction of cilia and emphasize mucosal preservation.

Senior et al. [7] showed the favorable long-term results of FESS, with 98.4% of 72 patients having improvement compared with before surgery over an average 7.8-year follow-up period. Although there was a steep initial learning curve, many studies have since highlighted the relative paucity of complications associated with the procedure. In a study of 250 patients undergoing FESS, Levine [8] reported that minor complications developed in 8.3% of patients, while major complications developed in only 0.7%. In comparison, a study of 670 patients undergoing the Caldwell- Luc procedure, the previous gold standard intervention for chronic maxillary sinusitis, showed a 19% major complication rate [9]. Finally, because FESS is based on a minimally invasive approach compared with conventional surgeries, there were less overall postoperative discomfort and shorter hospital stays.

Although FESS initially established itself as a less invasive, more targeted, and more effective technique than its predecessors, conventional FESS has evolved beyond this description. Originally, proponents emphasized that FESS provides a conservative and effective surgical intervention, rarely requiring a middle meatal antrostomy or stripping of diseased nasal mucosa. However, over time, there has been a departure from these conservative principles, with a tendency toward more aggressive intervention. As a result, surgeons have excessive freedoms in the nose, and sinus procedures are not standardized.

Although endoscopy offered a window for more precise visualization of nasal pathology, advances in other sinus instrumentation lagged. The original instruments used in FESS offered minimal precision, were associated with shear damage to normal mucosal tissue, and caused inadvertent stripping of mucus membranes. Technologic breakthroughs, coupled with a surgical model based on Messerklinger's principles [1], led to the next major advance in rhinology: powered instrumentation and the minimally invasive sinus technique (MIST).

DISCUSSION

Since its introduction in the literature in 1994 [9-10], MIST has grown in popularity worldwide. In the 2002, the first formal outcome study that compare MIST to FESS was published [11]. This study used the Chronic Sinusitis Survey (CSS) as the quality of life out-come instrument to assess improvement after MIST.

The outcome from MIST as measured by the CSS medication, CSS symptom, and CSS total subscales either equaled or surpassed those after FESS; the follow-up period for the MIST study was 23 months compared with 12 months of FESS and the surgical revision rate after MIST was 5.9% compared with an average of 10% after FESS. Furthermore, the results seen after MIST were consistent across the spectrum of disease severity (using CT grades I-IV), disproving the opinion that the procedure was only effective for minimal disease. These findings strongly support the recommendation that MIST be considered the initial surgical intervention for the treatment of chronic sinusitis. It strongly suggests that an excellent quality of life for chronic sinus sufferers could be achieved with minimal surgical manipulation of the nose and sinuses, it validates Messerklinger's transition space theory [1] and the reversibility of diseased nasal membranes, and it contradicts the rationale for the routine creation of a middle meatal antrostomy.

In fact, creation of a middle meatal antrostomy is occasionally required. Absolute indications include the biopsy of an antral mass, presence of ≥ 1 accessory ostia leading to maxillary recirculation, resection of a maxillary sinus fungal ball or inverted papilloma, and to allow for the application of topical medications or outpatient antral lavage in select cases. The concern with creation of a middle meatal antrostomy is not whether it works but whether it is necessary. Silva et al. [12] recently reported their study in which, for every surgical candidate with chronic rhinosinusitis, they performed a middle meatal antrostomy on one maxillary sinus but not the other. The results show no difference in the postoperative control of maxillary sinus symptoms or disease between the 2 sides. Thus, the potential risks of increased middle meatal scarring, interruption of mucociliary clearance and improper ostial function, development of maxillary recirculation by not including the natural ostia in the middle meatal antrostomy, and the likely need for revision maxillary surgery preclude the routine creation of a middle meatal antrostomy. Furthermore, authors conclude that the proper size of a middle meatal antrostomy can't be establish. Turbinate tissue is critical to proper nasal and sinus physiology. Routine resection of the middle turbinate often leads to edema and/or stenosis of the nasofrontal duct, and can produce compensatory glandular hypertrophy of the remaining nasal tissue. Powered shaving (i.e., thinning) of the lateral aspect of the middle turbinate and powered resection of the lateral wall of concha bullosa, including the natural bullosa ostium, can each improve middle meatal airflow without incurring the risks associated with turbinate resection.

Another, less formal outcome study on MIST titled "Minimally Invasive Sinus Surgery in the Geriatric Patient" was published in 2001 [13]. The study used a geriatric population (ages 65 - 93 years) of 100 patients undergoing MIST for chronic sinusitis, to assess whether, because of their age, they had a higher potential for intraoperative or postoperative complications. The study patients also assessed subjectively the quality of life outcome after surgery, 6 months postoperatively. Of patients, 84%

reported feeling significantly better, 10% somewhat better, and 6% unchanged. In comparison, another study of 119 patients with chronic sinusitis showed that 80.2% of patients had relief after FESS. Interestingly, 8 of 10 patients who reported feeling "somewhat better" after MIST, and 2 of 6 who had no improvement, had previously undergone aggressive FESS elsewhere.

The study also assessed whether there was any exacerbation of preexisting medical conditions or an increase in surgical morbidity after MIST. The 100 patients presented a spectrum of preexisting medical conditions, including hypertension, coronary disease, gastrointestinal disorders, diabetes, bronchitis and asthma, thyroid disorders, gout, stroke, renal disease, prostate disease, dysrhythmias, and others. Verifying the efficacy of MIST for the treatment of chronic sinusitis, the results highlight the fact that minimal medical/surgical morbidity is experienced by geriatric patients after MIST, making the procedure equally safe for the oldest and potentially most frail portion of the population.

A more recent article evaluated the efficacy of various middle meatal stents used during MIST [14]. Retention time for the Gelfilm stent was 5 days, whereas it was closer to 8 days for MeroGel, which is a statistically significant difference. Visible middle meatal synechiae on the right side (Gelfilm) developed in 4 patients, and none were seen on the left. The perioperative morbidity associated with the use of stents was negligible and not side specific. Mero- Gel appeared to be an excellent middle meatal spacer during sinus surgery. Compared with the literature, in which the rates of middle meatal synechiae vary from 27% to 4%, the overall synechia rate in this study was only 2% (0% for the MeroGel side).

A rationale has been provided for the aggressive ethmoidectomy now seen in contemporary FESS, however, to our knowledge, the basis for it remains unproven. It has been shown in both animal and human studies that osteitis of ethmoid [15, 16] serves as a nidus for recurrent infection or mucosal inflammation and, therefore, may be responsible for persistent/ recurrent disease after medical/surgical intervention. Thus, it is proposed that aggressive removal of all ethmoid sinus partitions will theoretically minimize the risk of recurrence.

Recent studies have shown that single-photon emission computed tomography bone scanning of the paranasal sinuses in patients with chronic sinusitis may be helpful in identifying foci of osteitis preoperatively [17]. These foci were correlated with histopathology of osteitis in 94% of cases examined. Therefore, CT absence of osteitis can address to MIST technique.

Regarding frontal sinus surgery, new mini-invasive approaches such as sinus balloon have been proposed. Currently the literature shows discordant results on this device so for our experience we recommend surgical approaches to this sinus with traditional surgery based on the principles proposed by Messerklinger to respect the sinus drainage paths [18]. About to the sphenoid sinus, we consider mini-invasive to carve the rescue flap to be repositioned on the spenotomy to prevent stenosis, iatrogenic mucocele and favor natural drainage [19].

REFERENCES

[1] Messerklinger, W.: *Endoscopy of the Nose*. Baltimore, MD, Urban and Schwarzenberg, 1978.

[2] Stammberger, H.: Endoscopic endonasal surgery–Concepts in treatment of recurring rhinosinusitis. Part II. Surgical technique. *Otolaryngol. Head Neck Surg.,* 94:147 - 156, 1986.

[3] Katsuhisa, I., Takeshi, O., Masayuki, F., et al.: Restoration of the muco- ciliary clearance of the maxillary sinus after endoscopic sinus surgery. *J. Allergy Clin. Immunol.,* 99:48 - 52, 1997.

[4] Asai, K., Haruna, S., Otori, N., et al.: Saccharin test of maxillary sinus mucociliary function after endoscopic sinus surgery. *Laryngoscope,* 110:117 - 122, 2000.

[5] Elwany, S., Hisham, M., Gamaee, R.: The effect of endoscopic sinus surgery on mucociliary clearance in patients with chronic sinusitis. *Eur. Arch. Otorhinolaryngol.,* 255:511 - 514, 1998.

[6] Min, Y. G., Yun, Y. S., Song, B. H., et al.: Recovery of nasal physiology after functional endoscopic sinus surgery: Olfaction and

mucocili- ary transport. *ORL J. Otorhinolaryngol. Relat. Spec.,* 57:264 - 268, 1995.

[7] Senior, B. A., Kennedy, D. W., Tanabodee, J., et al.: Long-term results of functional endoscopic sinus surgery. *Laryngoscope,* 108:151 - 157, 1998.

[8] Levine, H. L.: Functional endoscopic sinus surgery: Evaluation, surgery, and follow-up of 250 patients. *Laryngoscope*, 100:79 - 84, 1990.

[9] Setliff, R. C. III, Parsons, D. S.: The "Hummer": New instrumentation for functional endoscopic sinus surgery. *Am. J. Rhinol.,* 8:275 - 278, 1996.

[10] Setliff, R. C.: Minimally invasive sinus surgery: Rationale and technique. *Otolaryngol. Clin. North Am.,* 29:115 - 129, 1996.

[11] Catalano, P. J., Roffman, E.: Outcome of patients with chronic sinusitis after the minimally invasive sinus technique. *Am. J. Rhinol.,* 17:17 - 22, 2003.

[12] Sireci, F., Nicolotti, M., Battaglia, P., Sorrentino, R., Castelnuovo, P., Canevari, F. R. (2017) Canine fossa puncture in endoscopic sinus surgery: report of two cases. *Braz. J. Otorhinolaryngol.*, pii: S1808-8694(17)30040-X. doi: 10.1016/j.bjorl.2017.03.001.

[13] Catalano, P. J., Setliff, R. C. III, Catalano, L. A.: Minimally invasive sinus surgery in the geriatric patient. *Oper. Tech. Otolaryngol. Head Neck Surg.,* 12:85 - 90, 2001.

[14] Sireci, F., Canevari, F. R. (2017) Mininvasive surgical approach in endoscopic sinus surgery: when, why and how?. *The Rhinologist,* 3:42 - 4.

[15] Kennedy, D. W., Senior, B. A., Gannon, F. H., et al.: Histology and histomorphometry of ethmoid bone in chronic sinusitis. *Am. J. Rhinol.*, 108:502 - 507, 1998.

[16] Sireci, F., Speciale, R., Gallina, S., Sorrentino, R., Canevari, F. R. Clarithromycin in the Management of Chronic Rhinosinusitis: Preliminary Results of a Possible Its New Use. *Indian J. Otolaryngol. Head Neck Surg.,* 2018 Mar.; 70(1):87 - 91.

[17] Catalano, P. J., Dolan, R. W., Shah, R., et al.: Correlations between bone SPECT scintigraphy and histopathology of the ethmoid bone in chronic sinusitis. *American Rhinologic Society*, May 2004.

[18] Koskinen, A., Mattila, P., Myller, J., Penttilä, M., Silvola, J., Alastalo, I., Huhtala, H., Hytönen, M., Toppila-Salmi, S. Comparison of intra-operative characteristics and early post-operative outcomes between endoscopic sinus surgery and balloon sinuplasty. *Acta Otolaryngol.,* 2017 Feb; 137(2):202 - 206. doi: 10.1080/00016489. 2016.1227476.

[19] Rivera-Serrano, C. M., Snyderman, C. H., Gardner, P., Prevedello, D., Wheless, S., Kassam, A. B., Carrau, R. L., Germanwala, A., Zanation, A. Nasoseptal "rescue" flap: a novel modification of the nasoseptal flap technique for pituitary surgery. *Laryngoscope,* 2011 May; 121(5):990 - 3.

In: Handbook of Surgical Procedures
Editor: Heather Gilbert

ISBN: 978-1-53614-580-9

Chapter 7

COMPLICATIONS AND THEIR MANAGEMENT IN ENDOSCOPIC SINUS SURGERY (ESS)

Federico Sireci[1,*], MD, Francesco Martines[2], Pietro Salvago[2], MD, Claudio Sbacchi[1], MD, Vincenzo Immordino[1], MD, Bruno Galletti[3], Giovanni Cimino[1], MD, Francesco Galletti[3], Francesco Dispenza[2], MD and Frank Rikki Canevari[4]

[1]ENT Section, ARNAS Fatebenefratelli Hospital, Palermo Italy
[2]ENT Section, Bio.Ne.C. Department, University of Palermo, Italy
[3]Department of Otorhinolaryngology, University of Messina, Italy.
[4]Department of Otorhinolaryngology – Head and Neck Surgery, University of Genoa, Genoa, Italy

ABSTRACT

Endoscopic sinus surgery (ESS) is one of the most commonly performed procedures in otolaryngology. ESS complications should be distinguished in minor and major based on the treatment they need and

---

* Corresponding Author Email: federicosireci@hotmail.it.

the permanent sequelae they can cause. Over the years it has gone from an incidence of complications in endoscopic surgery of 8% for the major and 21% for the minor to a percentage of 0 -1.5% and 1.1-20.8%, respectively. This is due to the considerable diffusion of the technique with a progressive increase over the years of the surgical experience but their presence help to educate otolaryngologists and patients about complication rates in ESS in a modern context. A complication occurs when injuries to anatomical structures defined in the literature "risk areas" are created. The surgeon must know and identify these areas because these are important land mark that guide our interventions respecting the anatomical boundaries.

The aim of this chapter is to describe principle complications and their management.

INTRODUCTION

"An undesirable, unintended and direct result of an operation affecting the patient which would not have occurred had the operation gone as well as could reasonably be hoped" [1]. This is the current definition of surgical complication. These are distinct and classified according to gravity in 5 degrees [2].

FESS complications should be distinguished in minor and major based on the treatment they need and the permanent sequelae they can cause (Table 1) [3, 4].

Over the years there has been an incidence of complications in endoscopic surgery of 8% for the major and 21% for the minor at a percentage of 0 -1.5% and 1.1-20.8%, respectively. This is due to the considerable diffusion of the technique with a progressive increase over the years of the surgical experience. Ramakrishnan et al. in a 2012 retrospective study of 63823 patients report the following percentages for major complications: 0.17% rhinoliquorrea, 0.07% orbital lesions, 0.76% massive hemorrhage with need for transfusion [4, 5]. Regarding the complications in pediatric age, they are negligible with percentages below 1%, especially if the synechia are excluded. [6].

Table 1. Classification of surgical complications according to Dindo et al.

Grade	Definition
Grade I	Any deviation from the normal postoperative course without the need for pharmacological treatment or surgical, endoscopic, and radiological interventions
	Allowed therapeutic regimens are: drugs as antiemetics, antipyretics, analgetics, diuretics, electrolytes, and physiotherapy. This grade also includes wound infections opened at the bedside
Grade II	Requiring pharmacological treatment with drugs other than such allowed for grade I complications
	Blood transfusions and total parenteral nutrition are also included
Grade III	Requiring surgical, endoscopic or radiological intervention
Grade IIIa	Intervention not under general anesthesia
Grade IIIb	Intervention under general anesthesia
Grade IV	Life-threatening complication (including CNS complications)* requiring IC/ICU management
Grade IVa	Single organ dysfunction (including dialysis)
Grade IVb	Multiorgan dysfunction
Grade V	Death of a patient
Suffix "d"	If the patient suffers from a complication at the time of discharge (see examples in Table 2), the suffix "d" (for "disability") is added to the respective grade of complication. This label indicates the need for a follow-up to fully evaluate the complication.

*Brain hemorrhage, ischemic stroke, subarrachnoidal bleeding, but excluding transient ischemic attacks.
CNS, central nervous system; IC, intermediate care; ICU, intensive care unit.

Table 2. Classification of complications of nasal sinus surgery

Minor complications	**Major complications**
Temporary (not to be treated)	*Treatable*
- Subcutaneous periorbital emphysema - Periorbital bruising - Dental and/or labial pain/paresthesia	- Orbital hematoma - Reduction of the visus - Diplopia - Epiphora (which requires dacryocystorhinostomy) - Bleeding that requires transfusion - Liquorrea - Meningitis - Brain abscess - Focal cerebral hemorrhage
Temporary (to be treated)	
- Symptomatic synechia - Epistaxis - Pranasal sinus infections	
Permanent	
- Pain/paresesia dental and lip - Loss of smell	*Not treatable*
	- Death - Blindness - Diplopia - Central nervous system deficiency

A complication occurs when injuries to anatomical structures defined in the literature "risk areas" are created. The surgeon must know and identify these areas because these are not actually such, but they are important points of reference that guide our interventions respecting the anatomical boundaries. At present the major risk areas are summarized by the acronym "CLOSE" (C = Cribriform plate; L = Lamina papiracea; O = Cell onodi; S = Sphenoid; E = anterior ethmoidal artery) [7].

To better understand the possible complications, we will avoid addressing them by referring to this acronym but we will describe the main FESS steps highlighting for each of these the possible risks.

UNCINECTOMY

During this maneuver the risk areas are two: the lamina papiracea and the lacrimal duct (Figure 1).

CT scan is important to study the lamina papiracea in subjects who have never undergone surgery or who have had facial trauma because they may present spontaneous dehiscences or protrusions of the orbital fat within the ethmoid or maxillary sinus.

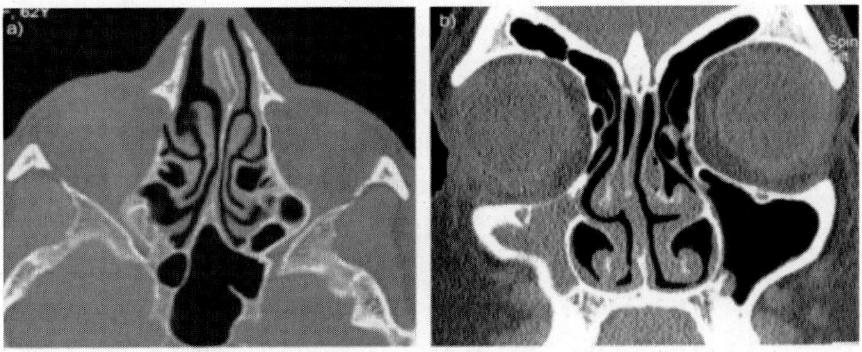

Figure 1. Risk areas during uncinectomy. The uncinate process is highlighted in red; in yellow the lamina papiracea.

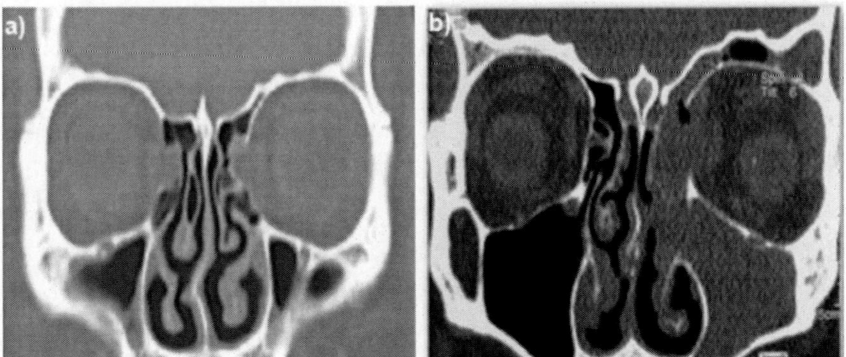

Figure 2. a) Spontaneous dehiscence of lamina papiracea; b) Lamina papiracea dehiscence in a patient with chronic rhinosinusitis.

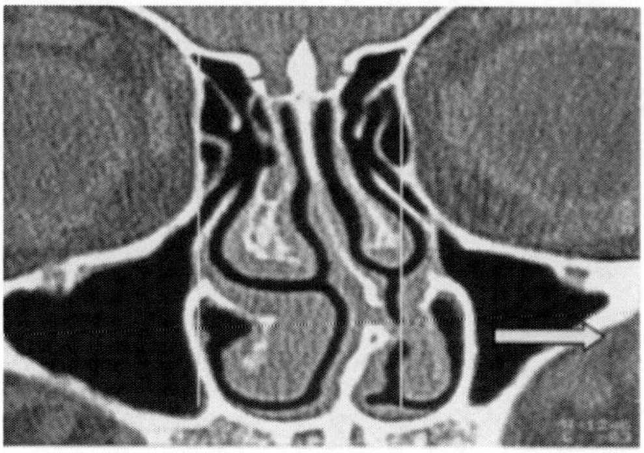

Figure 3. Medial wall of the maxillary sinus very lateralized with respect to the lamina papiracea.

Important is the evaluation of the projection of the medial wall of the orbit on the medial wall of the maxillary sinus. If the medial wall of the maxillary sinus is lateralized respect to the orbit (as in the "Silent Sinus Syndrome"), the uncinate process will be horizontalized, lateralized and leaning against the lamina papiracea. In these cases, during the uncinectomy, a downward correction of the backbiting forceps is necessary to avoid damaging the papyracea lamina and entering the orbital environment through the inferior-medial angle of the orbit.

Intraoperative safety measures are the execution of the Stankiewicz maneuver that allows us to evaluate infractions of the lamina papiracea and the use of the debrider with a tangential direction respect to orbit in order to prevent the aggression of endoorbitary structures. The use of the scalpel to dissect the uncinate process is by now a disused technique because it increases the risk of violating the orbital environment. Nasolacrimal duct lesion is a rare complication not reported in the latest cases because the hardest consistency of nasolacrimal bone is easily perceived by the operator. However, if it should be damaged, it is important to perform a dacryocystorhinostomy (DCR) intraoperatively to ensure proper drainage of lacrimal secretions. An untreated nasolacrimal duct lesion manifests clinically in the immediate postoperative period but in these cases a follow-up of some months (3-6 months) is recommended because often the epiphora resolves spontaneously. Only in 15% of cases can it occur even after the postoperative period [8, 9].

MIDDLE ANTROSTOMY

In addition to the risk areas described for the uncinectomy, it is possible to damage the sphenopalatine artery. This artery emerges from the sfenopalatin foramen delimited by the orbital process and the sphenoid process of the palatal bone placed in the posteromedial corner of the maxillary sinus. Therefore it is important to have an appropriate equipment (dessy bipolar forceps). The sphenopalatine artery and its septal branch vascularizes the posterior portion of the nasal septum that can be used as a closing flap in the skull base surgery, therefore it is desirable to preserve them. In surgical procedures within the maxillary sinus, other risk areas are the maxillary artery behind posterior wall of the maxillary sinus, the infrorbital nerve (V2) that runs in the median portion of the orbital floor and the superior alveolar nerve on the floor of maxillary sinus [10, 11, 12].

FRONTAL SINUS

The risk areas are represented by the anterior ethmoid artery and the lateral lamella of the lamina cribra.

The anterior ethmoid artery is a branch of the ophthalmic artery that runs from the orbit to the endocranium passing through the ethmoid roof. Anatomical studies on cadaver evidenced that in 91% of cases it is located inside the cranial base, therefore protected by the bone structure, while in 9% of cases it runs inside a mesentery suspended below the cranial base and therefore it is partial or total dehiscence [13].

The artery runs behind the first ethmoid foveola and often is protected by the cranial portion of the ethmoid bulla therefore frontal recess can be opened without decomposing the bulla can represent a measure of safety. The lesion of this artery can lead to an early intra or post-operative bleeding or to a massive intraorbitary bleeding with suffering of the optic nerve. For this reason, in the surgery of the frontal recess, the use of sharp instruments is recommended. In case of direct lesion of the anterior ethmoidal artery, it is sufficient to cauterize it with a bipolar forceps, possibly with a three or four-handed operation to maintain cleaned operating field, allowing an optimal visualization of the bleeding point. If the artery is retracted into an orbit by causing an intra-orbital hematoma, a lateral cantotomy of urgency can prevent the loss of visual function.

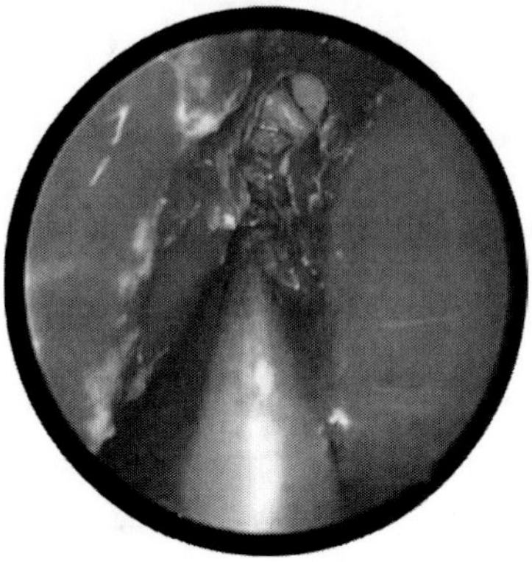

Figure 4. Dehiscent anterior ethmoidal artery in the left nasal fossa.

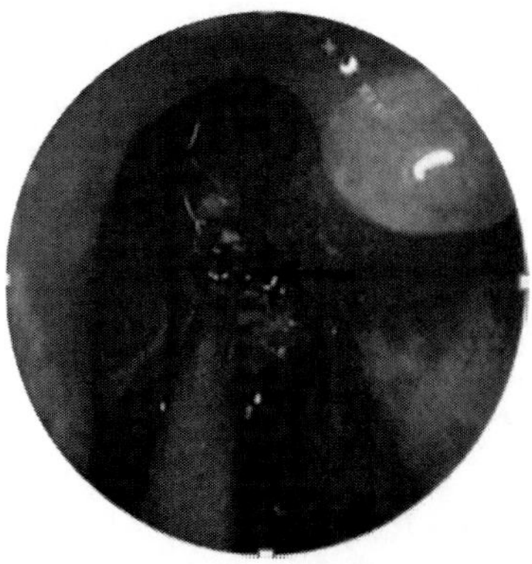

Figure 5. Rhinoliquoral fistula on the roof of the right nasal fossa ethmoid.

The lateral lamina of the cribra is very thin and in this area the dura mater is adherent to the periosteum so that a minimal bone infraction causes a tear of the dura with consequent rhinoliquorrea. In the preoperative planning it is important to evaluate the orientation and the length of the lateral lamina. Keros proposed an anatomical classification that measures the height of the lamina itself respect to the ethmoidal fovea determining so the depth of the olfactory fossa. There are 3 type: Keros I (1-3 mm) present in 12%; Keros II (3-7 mm) present in 70% and Keros III (7-16 mm) present in 18% [13]. A very long lateral lamina with a deep olfactory fossa increase surgical risk. Another parameter to be evaluated is the anatomical orientation of the lamina itself: if the lateral lamina is in a horizontal position, greater is the risk of CSF. It should also be noted that in 12% of patients there is an asymmetry between the two sides of 2 mm and that in about 6% of cases there are spontaneous dehiscences of the ethmoid roof [13]. In the frontal recess surgery safety measures are keeping intact, if possible, the ethmoid bulla, the use of sharp instruments and the execution of maneuvers from posterior to anterior and from medial to lateral.

If a CSF occurs, it must be recognized and repaired immediately in order to avoid further complications such as meningitis and/or pneumoencephaly. The administration of intrathecal fluorescein, useful in the exact topodiagnosis of a fistula, is not necessary if the diagnosis of the complication is intraoperative while it is advisable if the diagnosis is post-operative. The repair of an iatrogenic fistula of the lateral lamina involves the isolation of the area of the liquorrea, the preparation of the area bordering the defect, demucosization of the surrounding areas, removing all the bony asperities in order to obtain a more homogeneous operative field and that allows the placement of the graft. The use of autologous grafts that allow a correct integration of the graft into the receiving site is preferable. For small fistulas (3mm) it may be sufficient to use an overlay technique using mucoperiosteal taken from the septum or middle turbinate. In the larger size fistulas a multilayer technique is used, regularizing the bone edges and using the muscular fascia (fascia or temporalis muscle fascia) to better activate the function of the fibroblasts. The use of biological glues is not to be considered a closing technique but can be useful in stabilizing the grafts using it as a glue of the edges of the same. Nasal packing with the purpose of supporting the grafts must also be avoided, because their positioning and/or removal can lead to dislocation of the grafts themselves. In the literature are also described cases of occult liquorrea with spontaneous resolution with a reported percentage of 3% [15].

ETHMOIDECTOMY

The anterior ethmoidectomy provides for the opening and removal of the ethmoid bulla after the breakdown of the uncinate process. The risk areas are laterally the lamina papiracea and above the anterior ethmoid artery and the lateral lamina of the lamina cribra. Papyracea lamina lesions may result in orbital complications. The appearance of post-operative orbitary ecchymosis is frequent. This complication does not compromise the orbital function and should be treated with the early nasal molding, the administration of broad-spectrum antibiotic and reminding the patient not to blow their nose for at least 20 days in order to avoid orbit emphysema. The presence of pneumorobita must be monitored because if it is stable it does not require further treatment whereas if it is evolving it may require the insertion of needles aspiration through the transpalpebral way to decrease the orbital tension caused by emphysema.

In case of exposure of orbital fat, it is recommended to refrain to reposition it to the endorbitary level and to limit the cauterization of herniated fat. Parameters that must be evaluated in case of orbital complication are the perception of the red color that indicate a lesion of optic nerve, the diplopia and the orbital pain of ocular movements, possible index of damage to the extrinsic orbital musculature. Safety measures in the decomposition of the bulla are its opening in the inferior medial angle, its subdivision in the medium lateral direction with sharp instruments and the use of the debrider with a tangential direction to the orbit itself.

Posterior ethmoidectomy involves the decomposition of the second portion of the basal lamina of the middle turbinate. The risk points in this case are the lower wall, the lamina papiracea, the ethmoid roof and the sphenoidal etmoid interface. Excessive removal of the inferior wall, formed by the third portion of the basal lamina of the middle turbinate, causes a destabilization of the middle turbinate itself which can lateralize and close the posterior ethmoid with the consequent formation of iatrogenic mucoceles. Regarding the lamina papiracea are worth the considerations made for the anterior etmoidectomy, remembering that the closer you get to the orbital apex, the more the medial rectus muscle approaches the papyraceae, thus increasing the risk of damage to the ocular muscles. The ethmoidal roof at the junction between posterior ethmoid and the sphenoid planum is frequently found in a lower plane with respect to the anterior etmoid simulating a sort of "hammock" stretched between these structures. The evaluation of the ethmoid roof trend must be made with the CT scans in sagittal projection in order to avoid a lesion of the ethmoid roof with consequent liquor fistula. Another possible site for complications at the ethmoid roof is the posterior ethmoidal artery. This usually occurs in a bone channel near the ethoidosphenoidal junction. One of his lesions is a rare occurrence. At the level of the ethmoid sphenoid interface the presence of Onodi cells should be evaluated. This is a cell of the posterior ethmoid, present between 4-42% of patients, which pneumatizes the supero-lateral face of the sphenoid sinus and may contain the optic nerve inside (4-8% of cases) and in rare cases the dehiscent internal carotid artery which are therefore at risk of injury during posterior ethoectomy [16]. The Onodi cell should be evaluated by comparing the three projections of the CT. Its incorrect evaluation may lead to optic nerve lesions and/or cataclysmic hemorrhages caused by internal carotid lesions.

Safety measures in the posterior ethoidectomy are its opening in the inferomedial angle of the second portion of the middle turbinate and therefore its decomposition in the first later lateral direction then using sharp instruments and making a lower correction in the decomposition of the most cranial portion. If surgical measures are required in the posterior portion of the posterior ethmoid it is advisable to first perform a sphenoidotomy to identify lateral and upper anatomical limits.

The surgical operations performed on the middle turbinate provide for a partial removal, for correction of a paradoxical curvature, a removal of its lateral component, in case of decomposition of a bullosa or subtotal removal, if the pathology to be treated requires the creation of large cavities. The risks in the treatment of turbinates are represented by its cranial insertion and its relationship with the olfactory shower. Torsion maneuvers can lead to a destabilization of the middle turbinate, which lateralizes in the postoperatrix, predisposing to the formation of mucocels or even causing a fracture of its cranial insertion with lesion of the dura mater and rhinoliquorrea. The section of the middle turbinate must always be conducted inferiorly to a line passing through the armpit of the turbinates (middle, upper and upper) so as to respect the lamina of the croissants seat of the olfactory mucosa. In the decomposition of the medium turbinate it is advisable to use sharp tools, the progressive decomposition of the same avoiding rough maneuvers and the respect of the lamina of the croissants keeping a lower level to the lamina itself.

SPHENOIDOTOMY

The sphenoidal sinus can be approached with two main approach: the direct paraseptal and the transetmoidal [17]. The common point of the two approaches is the identification and enlargement of the natural sphenoid sinus ostium. A non-natural sphenoid opening may expose the optic nerve to damage because the anterior wall of the sphenoid is inserted laterally and perpendicular to the orbital apex. This perpendicular insertion may determine, in case of fracture at its insertion point, an injury to the orbital apex by the insertion of bone spicules. The finding of the natural ostium provides further security of the surgical maneuvers in the presence of Onodi cells.

In the direct paraseptal transnasal approach, the landmarks are represented from the choanal border, then continuing vertically and medially to the tail of the middle turbinate, the tail of the superior and superior turbinate. The natural ostium of the breast is located at the top of the upper turbinate. This, depending on the pneumatization of the sphenoidal rostrum, can be felt in a medial position, and therefore directly visible, or in a more lateral position, hidden from the tail of the upper turbinate itself. The risk points in this approach are the posterior portion of the olfactory area and the sepal branch of the sphenopalatine artery on the anterior wall of the sphenoid itself. A lesion of the olfactory area may result in alterations in the olfactory function and if the anatomical disorientation continues, a lesion of the skullbase with consequent rhinoliquorrea. A lesion of the sepal branch of the sphenopalatine artery leads to a hemorrhage of simple control but compromises the vascularization of septal flaps useful in the reconstruction of the cranial base. Safety measures are the finding of the natural sphenoid sinus ostium maintaining a direction of the instruments parallel to the plane of the nasal floor and the visualization of the axilla of the superior turbinate that identifies the olfactory area. The septal branches start in an area that moves from the lower portion of the upper turbinate to the upper portion of the middle turbinate tail. Their preservation can be achieved by limiting the sphenoidotomy to an upper plane with respect to the vascular area or, if necessary a wider sphenoidotomy, looking for the subperiosteal plane of the anterior wall of the sphenoid and by detaching the mucoperiosteal in caudal direction exposing the bone wall which at this point it can be removed up to the coanal edge, preserving the vascularization.

In transetmoidal way, the landmarks are, after the opening of the posterior ethmoid, represented in sequence by the body of the superior turbinate, by its tail and then by the natural ostium of the sphenoid sinus. The superior turbinate is to be found in the medial and inferior potion of the most anterior portion of the posterior ethmoid. Once the upper turbinate body has been identified, it continues in its progressive section up to the finding of the natural sphenoid ostium. The risk areas are the same as those of the transnasal route (olfactory area and the septal branch of the sphenoplatin artery). Safety measures are the finding of the middle turbinate axilla that indicates the olfactory region, the correction of the section plane in caudal direction parallel to the nasal floor. The insertion of a curved instrument at the level of the sphenoethmoid recess and its finding by transethmoidal way provides us with a further security of the correct finding of the superior turbinate and of the ethmoidal sphenous recess.

The sphenoid sinus has a wide variability of its pneumatization. The risk areas are represented by the anatomical structures of the neighboring regions that imprint, more or less clearly, the profiles of the walls of the sphenoid. The most critical area is represented by the lateral wall where the internal carotid artery and the optic nerve run. These can be dehiscent and therefore more exposed to iatrogenic lesions [18, 19, 20, 21]. For a correct anatomical orientation it is necessary to identify the intrasphenoidal points of recognition which indicate the position of the confined anatomical structures.

References

[1] Sokol DK, Wilson J. (2008). What is a surgical complication? *World J Surg*. 32(6):942-4.

[2] Dindo D, Clavien PA. (2008). What is a surgical complication? *World J Surg*. 32(6):939-41.

[3] Re M, Gioacchini FM, Pasquini E. (2013). Il rischio professionale nella chirurgia endoscopica nasosinusale. In: *Torgraf eds. Il rischio professionale clinico-assistenziale in otorinolaringoiatria*. 435-459. [Occupational risk in nasosinus endoscopic surgery. In: Torgraf eds. *Clinical-care professional risk in otorhinolaryngology*]

[4] Sireci F, Speciale R, Sorrentino R, Turri-Zanoni M, Nicolotti M, Canevari FR. (2016). Nasal packing in sphenopalatine artery bleeding: therapeutic or harmful? *Eur Arch Otorhinolaryngol*.

[5] Ramakrishnan VR, Kingdom TT, Nayak JV, Hwang PH, Orlandi RR. (2012). Nationwide incidence of major complications in endoscopic sinus surgery. *Int Forum Allergy Rhinol*. 2(1):34-9.

[6] Chan KH, Kraai TL, Richter GT, Wetherall S, Todd JK. (2009). Toxic shock syndrome and rhinosinusitis in children. *Arch Otolaryngol Head Neck Surg*. 135(6):538-42.

[7] Weitzel EK, Floreani S, Wormald PJ. (2008). Otolaryngologic heuristics: a rhinologic perspective. *ANZ J Surg*. 78(12):1096-9.

[8] Bolger WE, Parsons DS, Mair EA, Kuhn FA. (1992). Lacrimal drainage system injury in functional endoscopic sinus surgery. Incidence, analysis, and prevention. *Arch Otolaryngol Head Neck Surg*. 118(11):1179-84.

[9] Sireci F, Canevari FR. (2017). Mininvasive surgical approach in endoscopic sinus surgery: when, why and how? *The Rhinologist.* 3:42-48.

[10] Sireci F, Dehgani Mobaraki P, Nicolotti M, Vitali M, Tomazic PV, Faralli M, Longari F Canevari FR. (2017). *Indications to Canine Fossa Puncture in Management of Maxillary Sinusitis: Review of Literature*. Cepal review.

[11] Sireci F, Nicolotti M, Battaglia P, Sorrentino R, Castelnuovo P, Canevari FR. (2017). Canine fossa puncture in endoscopic sinus surgery: report of two cases. *Brad J Otorhinolaryngol.* pii: S1808-8694(17)30040-X. doi: 10.1016/j.bjorl.2017.03.001.

[12] Martines F, Salvago P, Ferrara S, Mucia M, Gambino A, Sireci F. (2014). Parietal subdural empyema as complication of acute odontogenic sinusitis: a case report. *J Med Case Rep.* 21;8:282.

[13] Moon HJ, Kim HU, Lee JG, Chung IH, Yoon JH. (2001). Surgical anatomy of the anterior ethmoidal canal in ethmoid roof. *Laryngoscope*. 111(5):900-4.

[14] Keros P. (1962). [On the practical value of differences in the level of the lamina cribrosa of the ethmoid]. *Z Laryngol Rhinol Otol.* 41:809-13.

[15] Bachmann G, Petereit H, Djenabi U, Michel O. (2002). [Measuring beta-trace protein for detection of perilymph fistulas]. *HNO.* 50(2):129-33.

[16] Dessi P, Moulin G, Castro F, Chagnaud C, Cannoni M. (1994). Protrusion of the optic nerve into the ethmoid and sphenoid sinus: prospective study of 150 CT studies. *Neuroradiology.* 36(7):515-6.

[17] Montana F, Salvago P, Dispenza F. (2018). Pleomorphic Adenoma of the Nasal Septum: A Rare Case Report of A 14 Year-Old Patient. *Euromediterranean Biomedical Journal.* 13 (06) 028–030.

[18] Sethi DS, Stanley RE, Pillay PK. (1995). Endoscopic anatomy of the sphenoid sinus and sella turcica. *J Laryngol Otol.* 109(10):951-5.

[19] Labadie RF, Davis BM, Fitzpatrick JM. (2005). Image-guided surgery: what is the accuracy? *Curr Opin Otolaryngol Head Neck Surg*. 13(1):27-31.

[20] Martines F, Salvago P, Ferrara S, Messina G, Mucia M, Plescia F, Sireci F. (2015) Factors influencing the development of otitis media among Sicilian children affected by upper respiratory tract infections. *Braz J Otorhinolaryngol.* pii: S1808-8694(15)00091-9.

[21] Galletti C, Cammaroto G, Galletti F, Camps-Font O, Gay-Escoda C, Bara-Casaus JJ. Dental implants after the use of bichat's buccal fat pad for the sealing of oro-antral communications. A case report and literature review. *J Clin Exp Dent.* 2016;8(5):e645-e649.

In: Handbook of Surgical Procedures
Editor: Heather Gilbert
ISBN: 978-1-53614-580-9

Chapter 8

SURGICAL CORRIDORS IN THE TRANSPHENOIDAL SKULL BASE SURGERY

Federico Sireci[1,*], MD, Giulia Danè[2], MD, Francesco Martines[3], Francesco Dispenza[3], MD, Francesco Galletti[4], Giorgio Peretti[5], Matteo Vitali[6], MD and Frank Rikki Canevari[5]

[1]ENT Section, ARNAS Fatebenefratelli Hospital, Palermo, Italy
[2]Department of Otorhinolaryngology-Head and Neck Surgery, IRCCS San Raffaele Hospital, Vita-Salute University, Milan, Italy
[3]ENT Section, Bio.Ne.C. Department, University of Palermo, Palermo, Italy
[4]Department of Otorhinolaryngology, University of Messina, Italy
[5]Department of Otorhinolaryngology – Head and Neck Surgery, University of Genoa, Genoa, Italy
[6]Neurosurgery Section, SS Antonio Biagio e Cesare Arrigo Hospital, Alessandria, Italy

[*] Corresponding Author Email: federicosireci@hotmail.it.

Abstract

Sphenoid sinus is very close to important and vulnerable structures of the skull base and therefore a delayed diagnosis and treatment can be potentially lethal. Endoscopic sinus surgery is a safe and effective technique that allows a direct route to the sphenoid sinus and therefore is considered the gold standard for the surgical approach to this region. Over the years, the indications for transnasal approaches in skull base surgery have extended in order to obtain an adequate resection of the pathology as with other conventional approaches, with a minor morbidity and an equal efficiency.

Many classifications, divided in base of intracranial pathology or intracranial anatomical landmarks, have been proposed to define the transnasal corridors in base of the localization through the middle cranial base. In this chapter, we propose a review of classification of transsphenoidal skull base approaches and show the main transnasal corridors to the sphenoid sinus based on the anatomical sphenoidal target and extension of pathology.

Introduction

Endoscopic surgery of the sphenoid sinus has been a great challenge in the past years for both otorhinolaryngologysts and neurosurgeons, because of the difficulty in performing surgical maneuvers in a deep space (sphenoid sinus) through narrow structures (nasal cavities).[1-3].

Otorhinolaryngologists have used the endoscopic techniques to replace the conventional "open" approaches since early '80s [4, 5]. Metson et al. reported in 1996 a direct approach to the sphenoid sinus thanks to the development of rigid nasal scopes and the evolution of the technologies [6, 28].

Jho et al. in the '90s proposed a pure endoscopic transnasal paraseptal approach for the treatment of pituitary adenomas [7]. In the early years of this experience, the corridor used was a direct transnasal approach from one or two nostrils [8-11].

The cooperation of multidisciplinary groups, the experiences in anatomical cadaveric endoscopic study and the improvement of technologies and endoscopic instrumentations have led to an extension of the surgical indications [12-17, 28-30].

In the last ten years, many classifications of transnasal corridors in skull base surgery have been proposed [18-23].

Extended sellar and parasellar endoscopic surgery needs a preoperative planning of the surgical corridor, and this planning should be based on the anatomical sphenoidal target.

In this chapter we propose a classification of the surgical corridors in the transsphenoidal skull base surgery, based on the anatomical subdivision of the sphenoid sinus into four regions

1. Nasal Corridors

In transsphenoidal skull base surgery, a wide exposure of the sphenoidal landmarks is required to avoid surgical complications.

There are three main surgical corridors to this region:

- Direct transnasal (paraseptal);
- Transethmoidal;
- Transethmoido-pterygoidal.

To simplify the approaches, we divide the sphenoid sinus into four anatomical regions: sellar region, lateral parasellar region, suprasellar region and clival region.

1.1. Direct Transnasal (Paraseptal) Corridor

This approach to the sella allows a rapid access to the sphenoid sinus by using the natural way of access to the sphenoidal ostium. When advancing tangentially through the nasal cavity, the first anatomical landmark is the choanal border. Then, proceeding vertically medial to the middle turbinate, the second anatomical landmark to seek is the tail of the superior turbinate. Sphenoidal ostium is located superomedially and dorsally to the tail of the superior turbinate. After its identification, the natural sphenoidal ostium is opened inferomedially using circular forceps, microdebrider or nasal drill.

When the natural ostium has a lateral position and it is not clearly visible, the access to the sphenoidal cavity is obtained with a transrostral approach: in this case, the anterior sphenoidal wall is drilled directly medially an superiorly the tail of superior turbinate in order to avoid lesions of the choanal branch of the sphenopalatine artery, then the removal of anterior wall of sphenoid sinus proceed superolaterally to reach natural ostium.

1.2. Transethmoidal Corridor

In this approach, the sphenoidal ostium is reached through the dissection of the ethmoidal cells. The surgical procedure begins with uncinectomy, antrostomy and ethmoidal bulla removal. The second step is the opening of the posterior ethmoid, after the identification of the second portion of the middle turbinate (an essential anatomical landmark). The access to the posterior ethmoid sinus is obtained penetrating the second portion of the middle turbinate in a medial and inferior position with a j-courette and then enlarging with circular forceps. The third step is the identification of the superior turbinate, this structure represents the medial wall of the posterior ethmoid. The natural ostium of the sphenoid sinus is at this point identified and widened through the dissection of the inferior portion of the superior turbinate in a tangential direction.

1.3. Transethmoido-Pterygoidal Corridor

The key point of this approach is the identification and the cauterization of two vascular structures: the sphenopalatine artery and the vidian artery. After a wide transethmoidal procedure, the approach continues with a partial resection of the middle turbinate and a wide posterior antrostomy. The subperiosteal dissection between the tail of inferior and middle turbinates allows to reach the origin of the sphenopalatine artery which is coagulated and then resected. The ablation of the posterior wall of the maxillary sinus permits the exposure of the contents of the pterygopalatine fossa and the consequent detection of the vidian canal with his coagulation.

At this point, a drilling of the base of the pterygoid and of the lateral part of basisphenoid is performed, in order to obtain a direct exposition of the lateral wall of the sphenoid sinus.

2. Sphenoid Regions

2.1. Sellar Region

The sellar region is delimitated inferiorly by the sellar floor, superiorly by the superior intercavernous sinus and laterally by the cavernous sinus.

The paranasal direct corridor is the preferred approach to reach this region. A bilateral procedure is recommendable in order to obtain an adequate anatomical space to permit a 3- or 4-hands surgical technique and therefore an easier control of surgical complications, as intercavernous sinus bleeding.

The approach is usually extended anteriorly with the removal of 1 cm of the posterior part of the nasal septum and inferiorly, by a subperiostal dissection, to the sphenoidal floor with the exposure of the T made by the union of the sphenoidal floor with the septal rostrum.

The transethmoidal corridor is preferred when the anatomical variations of the ethmoid sinus decrease the anatomical spaces, or in case of a necessary extension of the approach to the medial part of the cavernous sinus.

A partial removal of the middle turbinate could be required to obtain a correct exposition of the sphenoidal floor.

2.2. Lateral Parasellar Region

The lateral parasellar region is delimitated medially by the medial part of the cavernous sinus, superiorly by the optic nerve, inferiorly by the vidian artery and laterally by the ethmoido-sphenoidal junction.

The surgical corridors to reach this region are the transethmoidal approach and the transethmoido-pterygoidal approach; this choice depends on the pneumatization of the sphenoidal sinus and of his pterygoidal recess.

In case of a non-pneumatized pterygoidal recess, a transethmoidal corridor permits an adequate view of the lateral parasellar region. Instead, in the presence of a pneumatization of the pterygoidal recess, a transethmoido-pterygoidal corridor is preferred, in order to have a direct view of the infero-lateral part of the sphenoidal wall.

In both corridors, a posterior antrostomy, a wide ethmoidectomy with the exposition of the lamina papyracea and a direct exposure of the optical apex is required. The corridors are completed with a controlateral direct paraseptal approach and a removal of 2cm of the posterior part of the nasal septum.

2.3. Suprasellar Region

The suprasellar region is delimitated inferiorly by the intercavernous sinus, laterally by the optic nerves and anteriorly by the ethmoido-planum junction.

In this region, a wide exposure is required in order to avoid complications in narrow anatomical spaces, in which many neuro-vascular structures are present.

The approach to this region requires a wide bilateral transethmoidal corridor with the removal of the middle turbinate and a direct exposition of the ethmoido-planum junction and of the orbital apex bilaterally.

Before the widening of the sphenoidal ostium, a septal flap is created (in accord with the Hadad procedure) in order to reconstruct the skull base defect.

2.4. Clival Region

The clival region is delimitated superiorly by the sellar floor, laterally by the carotid arteries, and inferiorly by the sphenoidal floor. The clival bone extends inferiorly in the rhinopharyngeal region.

The preferred corridor for the clival region is a bilateral direct paraseptal corridor, in this case a drilling of the sphenoidal floor between the two vidian artery (from the "T" to the clival region) is performed. A removal of 2 cm of the posterior part of the nasal septum (from the sphenoidal floor to the inferior choanal region) is required to adequately expose this region.

This corridor can be extended inferiorly with a rhinopharyngeal procedure, in order to expose the inferior clival region.

DISCUSSION

During last years, transnasal surgical approaches to the sphenoid sinus have been a great challenge for surgeons, because of the difficulty to adequately visualize a deep anatomical region and of the presence of important anatomical structures in contact with the sphenoidal walls [24, 25].

For many years, the most popular technique has been the sublabial transeptal approach, while other authors reported transethmoidal and transpalatal routes [26, 27].

The experience in endoscopic sinus surgery (ESS) and anatomical endoscopic studies have permitted to extend such approaches from a simple opening of the sphenoid sinus (i.e., during transnasal procedure for inflammatory disease) to the endoscopic surgery of sphenoid sinus for the removal of benign tumors [3-6, 28-32]. Then, the transsphenoidal approaches were proposed for skull base surgery.

Since Jho in early 1990 described his experience in endoscopic approach to the sellar region, transsphenoidal surgery had a fast development [7, 9, 10, 11, 13, 33, 34]. Growing experiences in endoscopic sinus surgery and the cooperation between Otorhinolarynglogysts and Neurosurgeons have led to an increasing interest in the transnasal endoscopic approaches to the middle skull base [9, 12, 15, 22, 23, 35].

Endoscopic skull base surgery started with mini-invasive targets, but nowadays is evolving, in order to obtain a good result with minimal access to permit an adequate resection, as with other conventional approaches [11, 14, 17, 19, 20, 36-38]. Evolving in skull base surgery required new closure strategies as multilayer closure and Hadad septal flap [16, 39-41].

In the last ten years, many classifications have been proposed, dividing the transnasal corridors according with the localization and of the extension of the pathology along the middle cranial base [11, 12, 18-22, 36-38]. However, there is a little consensus nowadays about the codification of the available approaches.

The best classification about surgical endoscopic transnasal corridors to the sphenoid sinus should consist of three types: trasnasal, transethmoidal and transethmoido-pterygoidal.

The difference in the extension and in the widening of the corridor depends on the anatomical sphenoidal target. For this reason, the sphenoid sinus can be divided in four anatomical regions.

References

[1] Cheung, D. K., Martin, G. F., Rees, J. (1992) Surgical approaches to sphenoid sinus. *J. Otolaryngol.*, 21: 1 - 8.

[2] Cakmak, O., Shohet, M. R., Kern, E. B. (2000) Isolated sphenoid sinus lesions. *Am. J. Rhinol.*, 14:13 - 19.

[3] Castelnuovo, P., Pagella, F., Semino, L., De Bernardi, F., Delù, G. (2005) Endoscopic treatment of the isolated sphenoid lesions. *Eur. Arch. Otorhinolaryngol.*, 262: 142 - 147.

[4] Stammberger, H. (1986) Endoscopic endonasal surgery-concepts in treatment of recurring rhinosinusitis. Part II. Surgical technique. *Otolaryngol. Head Neck Surg.*, 94: 147 - 156.

[5] Wigand, M. E. (1981) Transnasal ethmoidectomy under endoscopic control. *Rhinology,* 19: 7 - 15.

[6] Metson, R., Gliklich, R. E. (1996) Endoscopic treatment of sphenoid sinusitis. *Otolaryngol. Head Neck Surg.,* 114: 736 - 744.

[7] Jho, H. D., Carrau, R. L., Ko, Y., Daly, M. A. (1997) Endoscopic pituitary surgery: an early experience. *Surg Neurol.,* 47(3):213 - 22; discussion 222 - 3.

[8] Bolger, W. E., Keyes, A. S., Lanza, D. C. (1999) Use of superior meatus and superior turbinate in the endoscopic approach to the sphenoid sinus. *Otolaryngol. Head Neck Surg*., 120: 308 - 31.

[9] Locatelli, D., Castelnuovo, P., Santi, L., Cerniglia, M., Maghnie, M., Infuso, L. (2000) Endoscopic approaches to the cranial base: perspectives and realities. *Childs Nerv. Syst.,* 16(10-11):686 - 91.

[10] Har-El, G., Swanson, R. M. (2001) The superiorturbinectomy approach to isolated sphenoid sinus disease and to sella turcica. *Am. Jour. Rhinol.,* 15: 149 - 156.

[11] Castelnuovo, P., Pistochini, A., Locatelli, D. (2006) Different surgical approaches to the sellar region: focusing on the "two nostrils four hands technique". *Rhinology,* 44(1):2 - 7.

[12] Cavallo, L. M., Messina, A., Cappabianca, P., Esposito, F., De Divitis, E., Gardner, P., Tschabitscher, M. (2005) Endoscopic endonasal surgery of the midline skull base:anatomical study and clinical considerations. *Neurosurg. Focus*, 15: 19(1):E2.

[13] Cappabianca, P., de Divitiis, E. (2004) Endoscopy and trans-sphenoidal surgery. *Neurosurgery,* 54(5):1043 - 48; discussions 1048 - 50. Review.

[14] Frank, G., Pasquini, E., Mazzatenta, D. (2001) Extended trasnsphenoidal apporach. *J. Neurosurg*., 95: 917 – 918.

[15] Frank, G., Pasquini, E. (2002) Endoscopic endonasal approaches to the cavernous sinus: surgical approaches. *Neurosurgery,* 50: 675 – 679.

[16] Locatelli, D., Vitali, M., Custodi, V. M., Scagnelli, P., Castelnuovo, P., Canevari, F. R. (2009) Endonasal approaches to sellar and para

sellar regions: clousure techniques using biomaterials. *Acta Neurochir.*, 151: 1431 - 7.

[17] Locatelli, D., Canevari, F. R., Acchiardi, I., Castelnuovo, P. (2010) The endoscopic diving technique in pituitary and cranial base surgery: technical note. *Neurosurgery*, 66: E400-1.

[18] Schwartz, T. H., Fraser, J. F., Brown, S., Tabaee, A., Kacker, A., Anand, V. K. (2008) Endoscopic cranial base surgery: classification of operative approaches. *Neurosurgery,* 62(5):991 - 1002; discussion 1002 - 5.

[19] Kassam, A., Snyderman, C. H., Mintz, A., Gardner, P., Carrau, R. L. (2005) Expanded endonasal approach: the rostrocaudal axis. Part I. Crista galli to the sella turcica. *Neurosurg. Focus*, 19(1):E3. Review.

[20] Kassam, A., Snyderman, C. H., Mintz, A., Gardner, P., Carrau, R. L. (2005) Expanded endonasal approach: the rostrocaudal axis. Part II. Posterior clinoids to the foramen magnum. *Neurosurg. Focus,* 19(1):E4.

[21] Couldwell, W. T., Weiss, M. H., Rabb, C., Liu, J. K., Apfelbaum, R. I., Fukushima, T. (2004) Variations on the standard transsphenoidal approach to the sellar region, with emphasis on the extended approaches and parasellar approaches: surgical experience in 105 cases. *Neurosurgery*, 55(3):539-47; discussion 547 - 50.

[22] Stamm, A. M. (2006) Transnasal endoscopy-assisted skull base surgery. *Ann. Otol. Rhinol. Laryngol.,* Suppl. 196:45 - 53.

[23] Castelnuovo, P., Dallan, I., Battaglia, P., Bignami, M. (2010) Endoscopic endonasal skull base surgery: past, present and future. *Eur. Arch. Otorhinolaryngol.*, 267(5):649 - 63. Epub 2010 Jan. 9.

[24] Rhoton, A. L. The sellar region. *Neurosurgery*, (2002) 51 suppl1: 335 - 374.

[25] Sethi, S. D., Stanley, R. E., Pillay, P. K. (1995) Endoscopic anatomy of the sphenoid sinus and sella turcica. *J. Laryngol. Otol.*, 109: 951 - 955.

[26] Spencer, W. R., Levine, J. M., Couldwell, W. T., Brown-Wagner, M., Moscatello, A. (2000) Approaches to the sellar and parasellar region: a retrospective comparsion of the endonasal-transsphenoidal

and sublabial-trassphenoidal approaches. *Otolaryngol. Head Neck Surg.*, 122: 367 - 369.

[27] Hardy, J. (1971) Transsphenoidal hypophysectomy. *J. Neurosurg.*, 34: 582 - 594.

[28] Setlif, R. (1993) The hummer. *Paper presented at the International Endoscopic Sinus Symposium*, Philadelphia, PA.

[29] Canevari, F. R., Giourgos, G., Pistochini, A. (2014) The endoscopic transnasal paraseptal approach to a sphenoid sinus osteoma: case report and literature review. *Ear Nose Throat J.*, 93(4-5):148.

[30] Vitali, M., Canevari, F. R., Cattalani, A., Grasso, V., Somma, T., Cavallo, L. M., Barbanera, A. (2017) High altitude exposure as possible predisposing factor for pituitary adenoma apoplexy: histologically confirmed case report. *J. Neurosurg. Sci.*, doi:10. 23736/S0390-5616.17.03987-X.

[31] Castelnuovo, P., Gera, R., Di Giulio, G., Canevari, F. R., Benazzo, M., Emanuelli, E., Galli, J., Di Girolamo, S., Staffieri, A. (2000) Paranasal sinus mucose. *Acta Otorhinolaryngol. Ital.*, 20: 6 - 15.

[32] Pagella, F., Giourgos, G., Matti, E., Canevari, F. R., Carena, P. (2011) Endoscopic treatment of maxillary inverted papilloma. *Rhinology*, 49: 369 - 374.

[33] Cappabianca, P., Cavallo, L. M., de Divitiis, O., Solari, D., Esposito, F., Colao, A. (2008) Endoscopic pituitary surgery. *Pituitary,* 11(4): 385 - 90. Review.

[34] De Divitiis, E. (2006) Endoscopic transsphenoidal surgery: stone-in-the-pond effect. *Neurosurgery,* 59(3):512 - 20; discussion 512 - 20.

[35] Maroon, J. C. (2005) Skull base surgery: past, present, and future trends. *Neurosurg. Focus*, 15; 19(1):E1.

[36] Cavallo, L. M., de Divitiis, O., Aydin, S., Messina, A., Esposito, F., Iaconetta, G., Talat, K., Cappabianca, P., Tschabitscher, M. (2007) Extended endoscopic endonasal transsphenoidal approach to the suprasellar area: anatomic considerations--part 1. *Neurosurgery,* 61(3 Suppl):24 - 33; discussion 33 - 4.

[37] Wang, Q., Lan, Q., Lu, X. J. (2010) Extended endoscopic endonasal transsphenoidal approach to the suprasellar region: anatomic study

and clinical considerations. *J. Clin. Neurosci.*, 17(3):342 - 6. Epub 2010 Jan. 13.

[38] Cappabianca, P., Cavallo, L. M., Esposito, F., De Divitiis, O., Messina, A., De Divitiis, E. (2008) Extended endoscopic endonasal approach to the midline skull base: the evolving role of transsphenoidal surgery. *Adv. Tech. Stand. Neurosurg.*, 33:151 - 99.

[39] Seda, L., Camara, R. B., Cukiert, A., Burattini, J. A., Mariani, P. P. (2006) Sellar floor reconstruction after transsphenoidal surgery using fibrin glue without grafting or implants> technical note. *Surg. Neurol.,* 66: 46 - 49.

[40] Hadad, G. Bassagasteguy, L., Carrau, R. L., Mataza, J. C., Kassam, A., Snyderman, C. H., Mintz, A. (2006) A novel reconstructive technique after endoscopic expanded andonasal approaches: vascular pedicle nasoseptal flap. *Laryngoscope,* 116: 1882 - 1886.

[41] Castelnuovo, P., Delù, G., Locatelli, D., Padoan, G., De Bernardi, F., Pistocchini, A., Bignami, M. (2006) Endonasal endoscopic duraplasty: our experience. *Skull Base*, 16: 19 - 24.

[42] Sireci, F., Speciale, R., Sorrentino, R., Turri-Zanoni, M., Nicolotti, M., Canevari, F. R. (2017) Nasal packing in sphenopalatine artery bleeding: therapeutic or harmful? *Eur. Arch. Otorhinolaryngol.,* 274(3):1501-1505. doi: 10.1007/s00405-016-4381-y.

In: Handbook of Surgical Procedures
Editor: Heather Gilbert
ISBN: 978-1-53614-580-9

Chapter 9

CANINE FOSSA PUNCTURE FOR THE MANAGEMENT OF MAXILLARY SINUSITIS

Federico Sireci[1], MD, Francesco Martines[2], Francesca De Bernardi,[3], MD, Salvatore Poma[4], MD, Francesco Dispenza[2], MD, Bruno Galletti[5], Francesco Galletti,[5] and Frank Rikki Canevari[6]

[1]ENT Section, ARNAS Fatebenefratelli Hospital, Palermo Italy
[2]ENT Section, Bio.Ne.C. Department, University of Palermo, Italy
[3]Department of Otorhinolaryngology, University of Insubria, Varese, Italy
[4]ENT Section, Villa Sofia-Cervello Hospital, Palermo Italy
[5]Department of Otorhinolaryngology, University of Messina, Italy.
[6]Department of Otorhinolaryngology – Head and Neck Surgery, University of Genoa, Genoa, Italy

ABSTRACT

Chronic rhinosinusitis (CRS) with nasal polyposis (NP) is a common chronic disease that often affects maxillary sinus. Endoscopic sinus surgery (ESS) is the most common procedure to treat the maxillary sinus lesions by a middle meatal antrostomy (MMA) and the introducing of new microdebrider blades of 15, 40, 70, and 120° improved this approach.

Nevertheless in some cases, angled microdebrider are not sufficient and canine fossa puncture (CFP) is performed as an alternative method to obtain a complete access to the maxillary antrum.

INTRODUCTION

Chronic rhinosinusitis (CRS) with nasal polyposis (NP) is a common chronic disease that seriously affects the quality of life [1]. The blockage of the ostiomeatal complex is the most common factor influencing the pathogenesis of this inflammatory proces [2]. Endoscopic sinus surgery (ESS) is the most common procedure for treating CRS that is refractory to medical treatment.

Although the majority of maxillary sinus lesions can be removed through the widened natural ostium performing partial uncinectomy and middle meatal antrostomy (MMA), some patients have extensive disease that is difficult to handle purely endoscopically.

In fact, endoscopic surgery of natural ostium allow to clear the posterior lateral wall, the posterior region of the roof, and the posterior wall of the maxillary sinus but no anterior and inferior regions. Failure to remove massive polyposis and fungal debris from the maxillary sinus may result in an early postoperative recurrence of symptoms and disease for the patient [3].

One solution is the traditional Caldwell Luc approach performed through the anterior wall of the maxillary sinus. However, this is associated with significant morbidity such as facial numbness or paresthesia (9%) for damage of the infraorbital and anterior superior alveolar nerves, oroantral fistulas (1%), gingivolabial wound dehiscences

(1.5%), and dacryocystitis (2.5%). This technique has been outdated by endoscopic medial maxillectomy useful to treat benign tumors, not inflammatory disease [4]. Canine fossa puncture (CFP) has been proposed as an alternative method of obtaining access to the maxillary antrum.

Although few studies have demonstrated the benefits of CFP in management of the severely diseased maxillary sinus, the efficacy and superiority of this method compared with conventional MMA, require further investigation above all considering new microdebrider blades of 15, 40, 70, and 120° that can be inserted through the antrostomy [5].

The aim of this study is to review the literature about the indications of CFP in patients with severe maxillary sinus disease and compare this surgical procedure with maxillary sinus clearance through MMA.

Canine Fossa Puncture Technique

CFP consist in a trocar placed in the canine fossa [6]. The landmarks in canine approach are: the mid pupillary line and horizontal line running along the lower border of nasal ala and lateral aspect of canine fossa high above the 3rd and 4th teeth (canine and premolar), infero lateral to infra orbital foramen. The trocar should be aimed towards the maxillo ethmoid angle to avoid pterygopalatine fossa and orbital lesions. In most patients the trocar was inserted using a gentle twisting motion. In some patients with thicker bone, gentle tapping with a hammer was required for the trocar to be inserted [7, 8]. After removal of the trocar a 4-mm microdebrider blade was placed through the passage created by the trocar. The microdebrider blade was visualized in the maxillary sinus with a 40 or 70° endoscope via the middle meatal antrostomy. Polyps and diseased tissue can be removed from the maxillary sinus using the microdebrider.

Discussion

Nowadays, middle meatal antrostomy (MMA) is considered the gold standard in the treatment of maxillary sinusitis. Anyway critical areas such as inferior, lateral, anterior wall, recessus zygomaticus and recessus alveolaris and recessus prelacrimalis of maxillary sinus are difficult to approach. For this reason, medial maxillectomy or external approaches such as Caldwell Luc approach or CFP are required [6].

The efficacy of this manoeuvre on the outcome after FESS has been investigated in few studies. Lee et al. have compared the results of performing a canine fossa puncture with clearance of polyps via a middle meatal antrostomy. No benefit of the canine fossa procedure over conventional middle meatal antrostomy was seen after 12 months follow up, however series are small in both groups (11 CFP V.S. 13 MMA). The authors concluded that although canine fossa puncture is a useful method for removing severe mucosal disease that cannot be reached through the MMA, it does not guarantee a better subjective or objective surgical outcome in patients with nasal polyposis [3]. However, Seiberling et al. in a case control studies have found that patients with the same disease who had a canine fossa puncture had a better outcome than those who did not. In fact, all patients were administered the chronic sinusitis survey (CSS) that evidenced a subscore better in the CFP group (Mann-Whitney test, P 0.02) [9].

In the last years, the advent of angled microdebrider blade (15, 40, 70, 120°) modified sinus endoscopic surgery allowing to reach critical areas of maxillary sinus but we have few references in literature that compare these instruments with CFP approach. Beswick et al. quantified the maxillary sinus volume and mucosal surface area (SA) that is accessible endoscopically via a middle meatal antrostomy in eight cadaver maxillary sinuses configured with image guidance software. In particular the authors demonstrated that mean maxillary sinus volume was 16.5 + 2.5 cm^3 and mean SA was 31.0 + 2.3 cm^2. The 15, 40, 70 and 120° microdebriders accessed an average of 10, 25, 41, and 66%, respectively, of the SA, and of 2, 9, 17, and 36%, respectively, of the volume. There was a trend toward improved accessibility of the superior half versus the inferior half of the maxillary sinus. When instruments of different degrees were combined to maximize accessibility, 81% of the SA of the sinus could be accessed. However authors did not quantify volume and area of maxillary sinus exposed [10]. Feldt et al. in a sample of cadavers showed that a significant greater amount of debris was left after the transnasal endoscopic technique (TN) approach compared with canine fossa trephination (CFT) (3.88 cm^3 vs 2.88 cm^3, $p = 0.015$). Median blade utilization was significantly higher with the TN approach vs CFT (4 vs 1, $p < 0.002$).

Therefore, although using new curved blades, critical areas such as antero-medial portion of MS cannot be reached and treated by antrostomy and therefore CFP has to be performed. According to literature, CFP can be performed only in unilateral lesions. In fact Byun et al. assigned randomly twelve patients to the CFP and thirteen to MMA groups who completed the follow-up, questionnaires (SNOT-20 and VAS), and postoperative CT evaluation. SNOT-20 and VAS scores improved significantly at 3, 6, and 12 months post-procedure in both groups. However, significant improvement of SNOT-20 at 12 months and VAS scores for purulent discharge, foul odor, and postnasal drip at 6 and 12 months were observed in the CFP group compared with the MMA group. Postoperative CT scan evidenced that the volume of mucosal thickening was significantly greater in the MMA group than in the CFP group. In addition, CFP was not effective in patients with bilateral CRS and diffuse NP but provided better management and subjective and objective surgical outcomes in patients with unilateral CRS accompanying NP 2. Among unilateral NP, there are anthrocoanal polyps (ACP). ACP is relatively unusual in the sinonasal tract. It occurs predominantly in children and young adults and originates from the maxillary antrum with extension into the nasopharynx or oropharynx. Simple excision of the polyp via limited surgical procedures such as simple polypectomy results in high recurrence rates. Complete removal of the polyp in the antrum, including its site of origin, is essential to minimize recurrence. However, a broad base such as a lateral, inferior, or anterior location of the polyp makes eradication difficult via a MMA. In this situation, some authors choose the traditional Caldwell-Luc operation, even in children [11]. However, the increased morbidity of this procedure, including facial numbness, facial swelling, risk for injury of the tooth buds and roots, and possible asymmetric facial growth, makes it less favorable than endoscopic sinus surgery. In fact, CFP is considered an alternative method of accessing almost the entire maxillary antrum in young/adult population. Few studies have reported the efficacy of the CFP approach in treating ACP in the pediatric population ($\leq$ 15 years old) and the long-term effect on changes in the maxillary sinus volume and surgical outcome has not been determined. Jae Yong Lee et al. studied a little sample of seven patients with ACP removed via the CFP approach. After a mean follow-up period of 43.9 months, the authors compared the changes in the maxillary sinus volume between the operated and normal sides, using the pre- and postoperative CT data. No contractures or decrease in the maxillary sinus volume on the diseased side were observed in any of the patients on postoperative CT. None of the patients showed evidence of recurrence on the endoscopic and CT examinations and only two patients complained of mild facial swelling and tingling sensation, which resolved spontaneously within 2 weeks [13]. Therefore, CFP can be performed to treat ACP in young but also in children when MMA is not sufficient.

Important indications to CFP are chronic odontogenic sinusitis (COS). Approximately 5–15% of the population suffers from chronic rhinosinusitis, and in 10–12% of them, it is of dental origin [13]. It is produced by periapical granulomas or small inflammatory cysts of the molars or bicuspids, chronic oroantral fistula (OAF), large odontogenic cysts occupying a great part of the maxillary sinus, and foreign bodies (dental fillings, teeth roots, and implants) pressed throughout the root canal or fistula into the antrum.

Venetis et al. presented 20 cases with odontogenic sinusitis, 5 (25%) in which a foreign body was removed from maxillary sinus by combined transnasal and canine fossa endoscopic approach. The surgical procedure was performed with conventional instrumentation through the widened antrorhinostomy or through a bony window at the anterior sinus wall. At the end of the procedure, the window was repositioned and stabilized with two to three absorbable sutures. In two cases, with sizeable foreign bodies, the preservation of the bony window was impossible, and a modified Caldwell–Luc operation was performed with preservation of the healthy sinus mucosa [14]. According to Barziliai et al. we avoid Caldwell–Luc operation because it is associated with significant morbidity such as facial numbness or paresthesia (9%) for damage of the infraorbital and anterior superior alveolar nerves, oroantral fistulas (1%), gingivolabial wound dehiscences (1.5%), and dacryocystitis (2.5%) [15]. Actually, Caldwell-Luc procedure is rational in cases of fungal disease and in endoscopic medial maxillectomy for treating inverted papilloma.

In the literature, different opinions about approach to fungal maxillar sinusitis are reported. In most of the patients it can be removed through the MMA using various curved instruments and saline irrigation without great difficulty. Also, if fungal invasion into sinus tissue is confirmed by histological examination, a systemic antifungal treatment postoperatively is paramount to reduce disease and potential recurrences [16].

Instead, there are no indications to perform CFP and/or Caldwell- Luc approach in maxillar sinus malignant tumor. According to the literature, endoscopic medial maxillectomy can be considered as first choice in difficult maxillary sinus tumor removal because an unnatural opening like CFA or Caldwell Luc in locally invasive disease with malignant potential as the tumor can extend through this opening in recurrent cases [17, 18, 19, 20, 21].

Conclusion

Although angled microdebrider improved endoscopic approaches to maxillary sinus, literature showed that canine fossa puncture is a minimally invasive technique useful in selected cases and without postoperative complications.

References

[1] Fokkens W, Lund FV, Bachert C, et al., (2005). EAACI position paper on rhinosinusitis and nasal polyp's executive summary. *Allergy*. 60:583–601. 2761.

[2] Sireci F, Dehgani Mobaraki P, Nicolotti M, et al., (2017) *Indications to Canine Fossa Puncture in Management of Maxillary Sinusitis*: Review of Literature. Cepal review.

[3] Lee JY, Lee SH, Hong HS, Lee JD, Cho SH (2008). Is the canine fossa puncture approach really necessary for the severely diseased maxillary sinus during endoscopic sinus surgery? *The Laryngoscope.* 118(6):1082-7.

[4] DeFreitas J, Lucente FE (1988). The Caldwell-Luc procedure: institutional review of 670 cases. 1975–1985. *Laryngoscope.* 98:1297–1300.

[5] Sathananthar S, Nagaonkar S, Paleri V, Le T, Robinson S, Wormald PJ (2005). Canine fossa puncture and clearance of the maxillary sinus for the severely diseased maxillary sinus. *The Laryngoscope.* 115 (6):1026-9.

[6] Anand V, Santosh S, Aishwarya A (2008). Canine fossa approaches in endoscopic sinus surgery - our experience. *Indian J. Otolaryngol. Head Neck Surg*. 60 (3):214-7.

[7] Petersen RJ (1973). Canine fossa puncture. *Laryngoscope.* 83 (3):369-71.

[8] Sireci F, Speciale R, Sorrentino R, Turri-Zanoni M, Nicolotti M, Canevari FR (2016). Nasal packing in sphenopalatine artery bleeding: therapeutic or harmful? *Eur. Arch. Otorhinolaryngol.*

[9] Seiberling K, Ooi E, MiinYip J, Wormald PJ (2009). Canine fossa trephine for the severely diseased maxillary sinus. *American journal of rhinology & allergy*. 23 (6):615-8.

[10] Beswick DM, Rodriguez KD, Olds CE, Kass JI, Schaitkin BM (2015). Quantification of maxillary sinus accessibility via a middle meatal antrostomy. *Am. J. Rhinol. Allergy*. 29 (5):394-6.

[11] Myers EN, and Cunningham MJ (1986). Modified Caldwell-Luc approach for the treatment of antral choanal polyps. *Laryngoscope*. 96:911–913.

[12] Lee JY, Baek BJ, Kim DW, Byun JY, Lee SW, Hong HS (2009). Changes in the maxillary sinus volume and the surgical outcome after the canine fossa puncture approach in pediatric patients with an

antrochoanal polyp: results of a minimum 3-year follow-up. *Am. J. Rhinol. Allergy.* 23 (5):531-4.

[13] Martines F, Salvago P, Ferrara S, Mucia M, Gambino A, Sireci F (2014). Parietal subdural empyema as complication of acute odontogenic sinusitis: a case report. *J. Med. Case Rep.* 21; 8:282.

[14] Venetis G, Bourlidou E, Liokatis PG, Zouloumis L (2014). Endoscopic assistance in the diagnosis and treatment of odontogenic maxillary sinus disease. *Oral Maxillofac Surg.* 18 (2):207-12.

[15] Barzilai G, Greenberg E, Uri N (2005). Indications for the Caldwell-Luc approach in the endoscopic era. *Otolaryngol. Head Neck Surg.* 132 (2):219-20.

[16] Pagella F, Matti E, Giourgos G, Colombo A, De Bernardi F, Castelnuovo P (2009). Is canine fossa access necessary for successful maxillary fungus ball treatment? *Rhinology.* 47 (4):385-8.

[17] Pagella F, Giourgos G, Matti E, Canevari FR, Carena P (2011). Endoscopic treatment of maxillary inverted papilloma. *Rhinology.* 49 (3):369-74.

[18] Sireci F, Nicolotti M, Battaglia P, Sorrentino R, Castelnuov P, Canevari FR. (2017) Canine fossa puncture in endoscopic sinus surgery: report of two cases. *Brad. J. Otorhinolaryngol.* pii: S1808-8694(17)30040-X. dei: 10.1016/j.bjorl.2017.03.001.

[19] Sireci F, Canevari FR. (2017) Mininvasive surgical approach in endoscopic sinus surgery: when, why and how? *The Rhinologist*, 3:42-4.

[20] Galletti B, Bucolo S, Abbate G, Canton Bascuas M, Romano G, Fera, G, Freni F. [Upper maxillary cysts: embryogenic and surgical considerations in our cases]. *Acta Otorhinolaryngol. Ital.* 2000;20 (3):177-86.

[21] Galletti C, Cammaroto G, Galletti F, Camps-Font O, Gay-Escoda C, Bara-Casaus JJ. Dental implants after the use of bichat's buccal fat pad for the sealing of oro-antral communications. A case report and literature review. *J. Clin. Exp. Dent.* 2016;8(5):e645-e649.

In: Handbook of Surgical Procedures
Editor: Heather Gilbert
ISBN: 978-1-53614-580-9

Chapter 10

POST-CRANIOTOMY TEMPOROMANDIBULAR DYSFUNCTION: PATHOPHYSIOLOGY, DIAGNOSIS AND TREATMENT

Thiago Martinelli, Fernando Akio Maeda, Claudio Fróes de Freitas and Andre Luiz Ferreira Costa*

Department of Orthodontics and Radiology,
University of City of São Paulo (UNICID), São Paulo, SP, Brazil

ABSTRACT

Several surgical procedures can be used to perform craniotomy, such as the classical pterional, pre-temporal and other fronto-temporal approaches. However, they are all based on the dissection of the temporal muscle, which can lead to temporal muscle atrophy, pain in the temporomandibular joint or masticatory muscles, weakness of the jaw closure, and development of signs and symptoms of temporomandibular joint dysfunction, all significantly compromising the patient's quality of life. This type of temporomandibular dysfunction has been frequently

* Corresponding Author Email: alfcosta@gmail.com.

neglected as only good results of the primary disease are considered. The following review presents a synopsis of the pathophysiology of post-craniotomy temporomandibular dysfunction and a practical approach to its evaluation and treatment.

Keywords: temporal muscle atrophy, risk factors, facial pain, temporomandibular joint, myofascial pain

INTRODUCTION

Orofacial pain can arise from a variety of disorders, including atypical idiopathic facial pain, temporomandibular dysfunction (TMD), dental pain, soft tissue diseases, neuralgia and headaches (Romero-Reyes & Uyanik, 2014). TMD is considered the main cause of pain in the orofacial region from odontogenic origin (Ahmad & Schiffman, 2016).

The aetiology of TMD is considered multifactorial, being comprehended in a biopsychosocial context (Manfredini, 2010; Marklund & Wanman, 2010). Although the prevalence of TMD changes depends on their pathology, it is reported that 75% of the general population have asymptomatic TMD (Costa, D'Abreu & Cendes, 2008).

The three cardinal features of TMD are orofacial pain, joint noise and restricted jaw function. Pain is the most common complaint and the primary cause for patients asking for help and treatment, thus being the principal goal of diagnosis and treatment (Manfredini, 2010).

As TMD is a musculoskeletal disorder affecting the temporomandibular joint (TMJ) and masticatory muscles, the pain exacerbated by the mandibular function is a pathognomonic sign of TMD (Kapur, Kamel & Herlich, 2003). It has been reported that nearly 50% of all TMDs are masticatory myalgias or masticatory muscle pain (Herb, Cho & Stiles, 2006). Myofascial pain and dysfunction of the masticatory muscles are more often stimulated by stress-related para-functional habits (i.e., clenching and grinding) (Herb et al., 2006).

TMJ pain from an articular disorder may conversely lead to myofascial pain (Herb et al., 2006). This is thought to happen due to reflex muscle contractions during mastication (Costa, Campos, Franca & D'Abreu, 2011; Okeson, 1985). Patients present with tenderness and hyperalgesia at sites distant from the joint, which may also include various trigger points (Herb et al., 2006; Murray & Peck, 2007).

It is known that any surgical incision in the masticatory muscles can affect their integrity, which, in turn, directly affects their function (Costa et al., 2014). Masticatory and cervical muscle disorders may result in changes in the mastication pattern, increasing the efforts of masticatory muscles, which may be followed by painful complications that could severely compromise the patient's quality of life (Costa et al., 2014; Figueiredo et al., 2006; Rocha-Filho, Fujarra, Gherpelli, Rabello & de Siqueira, 2007; Yasuda et al., 2010). Therefore, the dissection of masticatory muscles may cause cosmetic and functional problems in the patiens (de Andrade Junior, de Andrade, de Araujo Filho & Carcagnolo Filho, 1998; Rocha-Filho et al., 2007; Yasuda et al., 2010).

A wide variety of brain pathology may require surgical intervention, with craniotomy being the most commonly used surgical access approach. Patients who undergo craniotomy to treat intracranial pathologies may suffer a severe limitation regarding maximum mouth opening and develop different degrees of pain in the masticatory muscles and TMJ function (de Andrade Junior et al., 1998; Figueiredo et al., 2006; Rocha-Filho et al., 2007; Yasuda et al., 2010).

A closer look at these patients, especially with clinical analysis methods, reveals negative consequences because of injuries to temporal muscle resulting from the surgical approach, including muscle atrophy due to direct harm, ischemia, inadequate muscle tension, or muscle denervation (Abdulazim et al., 2012; Rocha-Filho et al., 2007; Yasuda et al., 2010). These post-operative side effects may arise after pterional and fronto-temporal craniotomy required in treatment procedures for refractory epilepsy, brain tumours or cerebral aneurysms (Yasuda et al., 2010).

Despite the increased awareness of the consequence of effective pain management following surgical procedures, an inadequate pain relief for post-craniotomy TMD still poses a significant clinical problem (Costa et al., 2014).

In this review, we focus on the primary research literature on the pathophysiology, diagnosis and treatment of post-craniotomy TMD for priority directions in reducing the associated complications.

PATHOPHYSIOLOGY

The pathological processes underlying the symptoms of post-craniotomy TMD involve the temporal muscle (Figueiredo et al., 2007) as its adequate function depends on proper innervation, vascularization, muscle tension and integrity of the muscle fibers. The functional integrity of the muscle requires a perfect innervation, an excellent vascular supply, muscle tension and inappropriate repair of the muscle at the site of original attachment (Kadri & Al-Mefty, 2004; Miyazawa, 1998; Oikawa, Mizuno, Muraoka & Kobayashi, 1996).

It is necessary an overview of the temporal muscle anatomy to better understand the pathophysiological data.

Muscle Components

The fan-shaped temporal muscle is composed of a central portion and three muscle bundles, namely, antero-medial, antero-lateral, and middle lateral (Kadri & Al-Mefty, 2004). The antero-medial muscle bundle is originated from the infra-temporal crest of the higher wing of the sphenoid bone, passing inferiorly and being inserted into the anterior region of the medial surface of the coronoid process and temporal crest. The antero-lateral muscle bundle is positioned on the lateral surface of the aponeurosis of the central part of the temporal muscle, and the cranio-medial region of this bundle is adjoined with the fleshy part of the temporal muscle. The middle lateral muscle bundle is observed as a thin sheet on the lateral surface of the temporal muscle aponeurosis in the middle region of its main part (Shimokawa, Akita, Soma & Sato, 1998).

Innervation

The anterior division of the mandibular nerve innervates the temporal muscle. This nerve frequently presents three branches: masseteric, middle deep temporal and buccal nerves. The anterior deep temporal nerve is a branch of the buccal nerve that can give rise to one or more branches. The buccal and anterior temporal nerves pass through the lateral pterygoid muscle, between the upper and lower heads of the muscle at its anterior aspect. Next, the anterior deep temporal nerve separates from the buccal nerve and divides into many tiny branches that supply the antero-lateral and antero-medial bundles, including the anterior part of the main portion of the temporal muscle (Kadri & Al-Mefty, 2004).

The middle and posterior deep temporal nerves run through the superior surface of the upper head of the lateral pterygoid muscle. The middle deep temporal nerve can originate separately or share a trunk with the masseteric nerve, which separates after leaving the foramen ovale, and innervates the middle part of the main portion of the temporal muscle and the middle lateral bundle. The posterior deep temporal nerve originates from the masseteric nerve as one or many tiny branches before it reaches the superior border of the upper head of the lateral pterygoid muscle, turning downwards to innervate the masseter muscle. The posterior deep temporal nerve supplies the posterior part of the main portion of the temporal muscle, with the masseteric and deep temporal nerves being related to the dorsal root of the zygoma (Kadri & Al-Mefty, 2004).

Vascular Components

In men, the blood supply to the temporal muscle is mainly derived from the anterior and posterior deep temporal arteries. There is an extra blood supply originating from the middle temporal artery, a branch of the superficial temporal artery (Cheung, 1996).

Effects of the Surgery on the Temporal Muscle

Alteration of the temporal muscle during neurosurgical procedures often results in tissue trauma, including fibre atrophy, presence of fibrotic tissue within the muscle, and reduction in muscle strength (Costa et al., 2014; de Andrade Junior et al., 1998; Rocha-Filho et al., 2007). Other abnormalities include cosmetic deformities (anterior temporal hollow) and functional handicaps (Kadri & Al-Mefty, 2004; Park et al., 2015). The post-operative sequelae of the temporal muscle may be originated from the following factors:

Consequences of Denervation

The return of motor function of a denervated muscle depends not only on the restoration of nerve supply, but also on the capacity of the muscle to respond (Wang, Gu, Xu, Shen & Li, 2001). After denervation, the skeletal muscle undergoes a sequence of morphological, physiological, biochemical, functional, and metabolic changes (Kadri & Al-Mefty, 2004; Wang et al., 2001). With prolonged denervation, the blood supply deteriorates and fibrosis progresses with ultimate replacement of muscle by fat tissue. All three deep temporal nerves are positioned superficially to the sub-periosteum and may be injured by dissection of the soft tissue. Therefore, sub-periosteal dissection is of vital importance in preserving the nerves (Kadri & Al-Mefty, 2004).

Consequences of Devascularisation

Muscular ischemia due to prolonged retraction or interruption of blood supply can produce irreversible damage after micro-vascular occlusion caused by propagation of thrombus, causing fibrosis and atrophy (Kadri & Al-Mefty, 2004; Miyazawa, 1998).

Integrity of the Fibres and Muscle Tension

Muscle tension is critical in conserving functionality and preventing atrophy from disuse (Kadri & Al-Mefty, 2004; Zager, Del Vecchio & Bartlett, 1993) as muscular attachments should be preserved to maintain the contraction of the muscle. Nevertheless, the injured fibres become fibrotic and present scars, thus harming the vascular and nerve supply to the distal part of the flap, which increases atrophy and asymmetry after surgery (Kadri & Al-Mefty, 2004). Preservation of the muscle fibres and restoration of the muscle alignment as similar as possible to that prior to surgery is crucial to minimise post-operative deformities of the muscle (Park et al., 2015).

Post-Craniotomy TMD

It has been shown that patients undergoing the same procedure for craniotomy may or may not develop muscle atrophy and/or TMD (Costa et al., 2014; de Andrade Junior et al., 1998). Dissection of the temporal muscle has an immediate effect, generating hypomobility caused by weakness and retraction of the TMJ muscles (Park et al., 2015). These factors can induce degenerative or adaptive changes in the joint tissue (Costa et al., 2014).

TMJ is often and intensively affected in patients who underwent craniotomy (Costa et al., 2014; de Andrade Junior et al., 1998; Rocha-Filho et al., 2007; Yasuda et al., 2010). It is interesting to note that the degree of joint impairment differs among these patients.

In post-craniotomy patients, many factors such as masticatory muscle weakness, dental malocclusions and bruxism can affect the dynamic balance or equilibrium between the components of the masticatory system (Costa et al., 2014). Bruxism is a non-painful disorder characterised as a repetitive jaw-muscle activity, such as clenching or grinding of the teeth and/or bracing or thrusting of the mandible (Lobbezoo et al., 2013).

Bruxism with undesirable occlusal patterns may lead to damage to joint tissues at molecular level, thus predisposing to joint intra-capsular dysfunction, joint effusion and pain (Costa et al., 2014).

In general, TMD can be influenced by concurrent myofascial pain and/or bruxism. Moreover, degenerative lesions in muscle fibers and inflammation after craniotomy can compromise the normal joint biomechanics, producing deleterious effects or degenerative changes in the TMJ (Costa et al., 2014).

DIAGNOSIS

The presence of concomitant bruxism is considered a risk factor for post-craniotomy TMD that can affect the surgical outcomes, being recognised as a causal agent involved in its initiation and/or perpetuation (Costa et al., 2014). Therefore, it is important that the physician determines the diagnosis of TMJ before surgery.

The diagnosis is clinical and uncomplicated, with evaluation being based on the patient's information, history and clinical analysis of TMJ. A TMD specialist can provide a global vision of the joint and mastication muscles by searching for pain/tenderness on palpation, joint noises, jaw function limitation, masticatory muscle pain, para-function habits (e.g., clenching, bruxism, nail biting) and anomalies of occlusal functions (Ahmad & Schiffman, 2016).

TREATMENT

Patients always present pain and mouth opening limitation during the first post-operative months (Yasuda et al., 2010), with the individuals showing gradual improvement over time. However, in some patients, symptoms may persist by reaching the joint and affecting structures (disc or cartilage) in the TMJ (Costa et al., 2014; Kadri & Al-Mefty, 2004).

Because the clinical presentation of post-craniotomy TMD is heterogeneous, the treatment should be individualised for each patient depending on pain severity, comorbidities, and level of functional impairment.

The management includes physical therapy to re-establish the mandibular function as soon as possible, with manual therapies (e.g., jaw exercises and re-education) being shown to be effective to reduce pain and recover mobility/function in the patients (Melis, 2013).

Manual therapy using soft tissue techniques, mobilisation, exercises and manipulation is proposed to reduce local ischemia, stimulate proprioception, break fibrous adhesions, generate synovial fluid production and reduce pain (Kalamir, Bonello, Graham, Vitiello & Pollard, 2012).

Active and passive range of motion exercises target to re-establish physiological movements by means of opening, laterotrusion, protrusion and retrusion movements have been shown to significantly reduce pain and injury, in addition to increasing the range of motion (Kalamir et al., 2012; Michelotti, Parisini, Farella, Cimino & Martina, 2000).

REFERENCES

Abdulazim, A., Filis, A., Sadr-Eshkevari, P., Schulte, F., Sandu, N., & Schaller, B. (2012). Postcraniotomy function of the temporal muscle in skull base surgery: Technical note based on a preliminary study. *ScientificWorldJournal,* 2012, 427081.

Ahmad, M., & Schiffman, E. L. (2016). Temporomandibular Joint Disorders and Orofacial Pain. *Dent Clin North Am,* 60(1), 105-124.

Cheung, L. K. (1996). The vascular anatomy of the human temporalis muscle: implications for surgical splitting techniques. *Int J Oral Maxillofac Surg,* 25(6), 414-421.

Costa, A. L., Campos, L. S., Franca, M. C., Jr., & D'Abreu, A. (2011). Temporomandibular disorders in patients with craniocervical dystonia. *Arq Neuropsiquiatr,* 69(6), 896-899.

Costa, A. L., D'Abreu, A., & Cendes, F. (2008). Temporomandibular joint internal derangement: Association with headache, joint effusion, bruxism, and joint pain. *J Contemp Dent Pract,* 9(6), 9-16.

Costa, A. L., Yasuda, C. L., Franca, M., Jr., de Freitas, C. F., Tedeschi, H., de Oliveira, E., & Cendes, F. (2014). Temporomandibular dysfunction post-craniotomy: evaluation between pre- and post-operative status. *J Craniomaxillofac Surg,* 42(7), 1475-1479.

de Andrade Junior, F. C., de Andrade, F. C., de Araujo Filho, C. M., & Carcagnolo Filho, J. (1998). Dysfunction of the temporalis muscle after pterional craniotomy for intracranial aneurysms. Comparative, prospective and randomized study of one flap versus two flaps dieresis. *Arq Neuropsiquiatr,* 56(2), 200-205.

Figueiredo, E. G., Deshmukh, P., Nakaji, P., Crusius, M. U., Crawford, N., Spetzler, R. F., & Preul, M. C. (2007). The minipterional craniotomy: technical description and anatomic assessment. *Neurosurgery,* 61(5 Suppl 2), 256-264; discussion 264-255.

Figueiredo, E. G., Deshmukh, V., Nakaji, P., Deshmukh, P., Crusius, M. U., Crawford, N., ... Preul, M. C. (2006). An anatomical evaluation of the mini-supraorbital approach and comparison with standard craniotomies. *Neurosurgery,* 59(4 Suppl 2), ONS212-220; discussion ONS220.

Herb, K., Cho, S., & Stiles, M. A. (2006). Temporomandibular joint pain and dysfunction. *Curr Pain Headache Rep,* 10(6), 408-414.

Kadri, P. A., & Al-Mefty, O. (2004). The anatomical basis for surgical preservation of temporal muscle. *J Neurosurg,* 100(3), 517-522.

Kalamir, A., Bonello, R., Graham, P., Vitiello, A. L., & Pollard, H. (2012). Intraoral myofascial therapy for chronic myogenous temporomandibular disorder: a randomized controlled trial. *J Manipulative Physiol Ther,* 35(1), 26-37.

Kapur, N., Kamel, I. R., & Herlich, A. (2003). Oral and craniofacial pain: diagnosis, pathophysiology, and treatment. *Int Anesthesiol Clin,* 41(3), 115-150.

Lobbezoo, F., Ahlberg, J., Glaros, A. G., Kato, T., Koyano, K., Lavigne, G. J., ... Winocur, E. (2013). Bruxism defined and graded: an international consensus. *J Oral Rehabil,* 40(1), 2-4.

Manfredini, D. (2010). *Current concepts on temporomandibular disorders.* London: Quintessence.

Marklund, S., & Wanman, A. (2010). Risk factors associated with incidence and persistence of signs and symptoms of temporomandibular disorders. *Acta Odontol Scand,* 68(5), 289-299.

Melis, M. (2013). The role of physical therapy for the treatment of temporomandibular disorders. *J Orthod Sci,* 2(4), 113-114.

Michelotti, A., Parisini, F., Farella, M., Cimino, R., & Martina, R. (2000). [Muscular physiotherapy in patients with temporomandibular disorders. Controlled clinical trial]. *Minerva Stomatol,* 49(11-12), 541-548.

Miyazawa, T. (1998). Less invasive reconstruction of the temporalis muscle for pterional craniotomy: modified procedures. *Surg Neurol,* 50(4), 347-351; discussion 351.

Murray, G. M., & Peck, C. C. (2007). Orofacial pain and jaw muscle activity: a new model. *J Orofac Pain,* 21(4), 263-278; discussion 279-288.

Oikawa, S., Mizuno, M., Muraoka, S., & Kobayashi, S. (1996). Retrograde dissection of the temporalis muscle preventing muscle atrophy for pterional craniotomy. Technical note. *J Neurosurg,* 84(2), 297-299.

Okeson, J. P. (1985). *Fundamentals of occlusion and temporomandibular disorders*. St. Louis: Mosby.

Park, J. H., Lee, Y. S., Suh, S. J., Lee, J. H., Ryu, K. Y., & Kang, D. G. (2015). A Simple Method for Reconstruction of the Temporalis Muscle Using Contourable Strut Plate after Pterional Craniotomy: Introduction of the Surgical Techniques and Analysis of Its Efficacy. *J Cerebrovasc Endovasc Neurosurg,* 17(2), 93-100.

Rocha-Filho, P. A., Fujarra, F. J., Gherpelli, J. L., Rabello, G. D., & de Siqueira, J. T. (2007). The long-term effect of craniotomy on temporalis muscle function. *Oral Surg Oral Med Oral Pathol Oral Radiol Endod,* 104(5), e17-21.

Romero-Reyes, M., & Uyanik, J. M. (2014). Orofacial pain management: current perspectives. *J Pain Res,* 7, 99-115.

Shimokawa, T., Akita, K., Soma, K., & Sato, T. (1998). Innervation analysis of the small muscle bundles attached to the temporalis: truly new muscles or merely derivatives of the temporalis? *Surg Radiol Anat,* 20(5), 329-334.

Wang, H., Gu, Y., Xu, J., Shen, L., & Li, J. (2001). Comparative study of different surgical procedures using sensory nerves or neurons for delaying atrophy of denervated skeletal muscle. *J Hand Surg Am,* 26(2), 326-331.

Yasuda, C. L., Costa, A. L., Franca, M., Jr., Pereira, F. R., Tedeschi, H., de Oliveira, E., & Cendes, F. (2010). Postcraniotomy temporalis muscle atrophy: a clinical, magnetic resonance imaging volumetry and electromyographic investigation. *J Orofac Pain,* 24(4), 391-397.

Zager, E. L., DelVecchio, D. A., & Bartlett, S. P. (1993). Temporal muscle microfixation in pterional craniotomies. Technical note. *J Neurosurg,* 79(6), 946-947.

Biographical Sketches

Thiago Martinelli

Education: DDS

Currently Master student in Dentistry program of UNICID – University of Sao Paulo City.

Fernando Akio Maeda

Education:

Associate professor of Master's degree program and Undergraduation Dentistry; UNICID – University of Sao Paulo City.

- DDS – 2005 - São Paulo State University - UNESP (FOA, Araçatuba, Brazil).
- MSc in Restorative Dentistry - 2009 - University of São Paulo – USP (FORP, Ribeirão Preto, Brazil).
- PhD in Dental Materials – 2010 - University of São Paulo – USP (FOUSP – São Paulo, Brazil).

Claudio Fróes de Freitas

Education:

Head of Master's degree program and Undergraduation Dentistry; UNICID – University of Sao Paulo City.

- DDS – 1986 - São Paulo State University - UNESP (FOSJC, São José dos Campos, Brazil).
- MSc - 1989 - University of São Paulo – USP (FOUSP, São Paulo, Brazil).
- PhD – 1991 - University of São Paulo – USP (FOUSP – São Paulo, Brazil).

Andre Luiz Ferreira Costa

Associate professor of Master's degree program and Undergraduation –Dentistry/UNICID – University of Sao Paulo City.

Postdoctoral Fellowship:

- Laboratory of Neuroimaging/Department of Neurology; Faculty of Medical Sciences; UNICAMP
- Department of Diagnostic Imaging/The Ottawa Hospital; University of Ottawa; Canada

Education:

- PhD program; Laboratory of Neuroimaging/Dept of Neurology; Faculty of Medical Sciences; UNICAMP
- Master of Dental Science degree (Oral and Maxillofacial Radiology); School of Dentistry, UNICAMP-(Piracicaba-SP, Brazil)

- Internship: Oral and Maxillofacial Radiology; School of Dentistry, USP-(Ribeirão Preto-SP, Brazil)
- DDS: School of Dentistry/USP-(Ribeirão Preto-SP, Brazil)

INDEX

C

D

E

F

G

H

I

L

M

N

O

P

Q

R

Pediatric Tonsillectomy: Intracapsular versus Extracapsular Techniques (DVD Included)

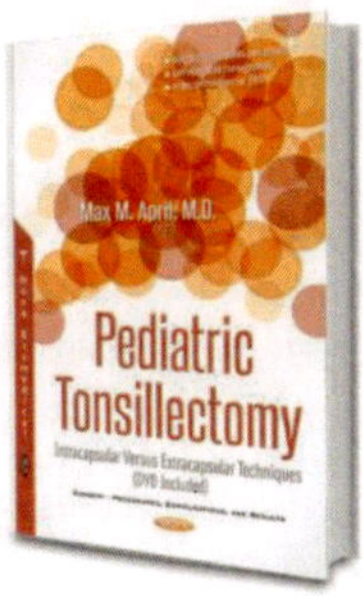

Editor: Max M. April, M.D. (Department of Otolaryngology, New York University/Langone Medical Center, New York, USA)

Series: Surgery - Procedures, Complications, and Results

Book Description: This will be a new type of surgical atlas describing not only basic techniques used in the beginning of one's experience but also more advanced maneuvers to improve results even further. Full length videos are included on a DVD.

Hardcover ISBN: 978-1-53612-706-5
Retail Price: $150

Advances in Experimental Surgery. Volume 2

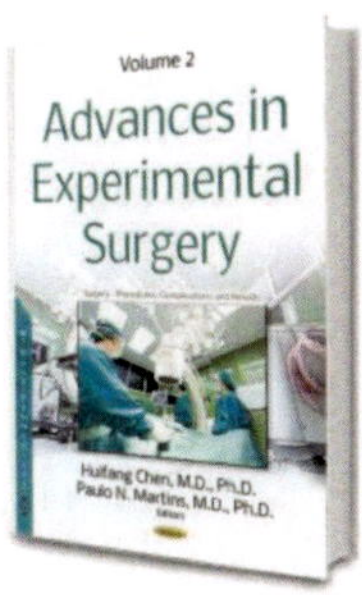

Editors: Huifang Chen, M.D., Ph.D. and Paulo N. Martins, M.D., Ph.D (Professor of Surgery, Laboratory of Experimental Surgery, Research Center, University of Montreal, Montreal, Quebec, Canada, and others)

Series: Surgery - Procedures, Complications, and Results

Book Description: This book documents the enormous volume of knowledge scientists have acquired in the field of experimental surgery.

Hardcover ISBN: 978-1-53612-773-7
Retail Price: $230